PERSONHO
CARE IN AD

Paul Higgs and Chris Gilleard

P

First published in Great Britain in 2016 by

Policy Press
University of Bristol
1-9 Old Park Hill
Bristol
BS2 8BB
UK
t: +44 (0)117 954 5940
pp-info@bristol.ac.uk
www.policypress.co.uk

North America office:
Policy Press
c/o The University of Chicago Press
1427 East 60th Street
Chicago, IL 60637, USA
t: +1 773 702 7700
f: +1 773-702-9756
sales@press.uchicago.edu
www.press.uchicago.edu

© Policy Press 2016

British Library Cataloguing in Publication Data
A catalogue record for this book is available from the British Library

Library of Congress Cataloging-in-Publication Data
A catalog record for this book has been requested

ISBN 978-1-4473-1906-1 paperback
ISBN 978-1-4473-1905-4 hardcover
ISBN 978-1-4473-1909-2 ePub
ISBN 978-1-4473-1910-8 Mobi
ISBN 978-1-4473-1907-8 ePdf

The right of Paul Higgs and Chris Gilleard to be identified as authors of this work has been asserted by them in accordance with the Copyright, Designs and Patents Act 1988.

All rights reserved: no part of this publication may be reproduced, stored in a retrieval system, or transmitted in any form or by any means, electronic, mechanical, photocopying, recording, or otherwise without the prior permission of Policy Press.

The statements and opinions contained within this publication are solely those of the authors and not of the University of Bristol or Policy Press. The University of Bristol and Policy Press disclaim responsibility for any injury to persons or property resulting from any material published in this publication.

Policy Press works to counter discrimination on grounds of gender, race, disability, age and sexuality.

Cover design by Soapbox Design
Front cover image: istock
Printed and bound in Great Britain by CPI Group (UK) Ltd, Croydon, CR0 4YY
Policy Press uses environmentally responsible print partners

My son, support your father in his old age, do not grieve him during his life. Even if his mind should fail, show him sympathy, do not despise him in your health and strength; for kindness to a father shall not be forgotten, but will serve as a reparation for your sins.

(Ecclesiasticus 3: 12-14)

Contents

Preface		vi
one	Old age and the fourth age paradigm	1
two	Interrogating personhood	11
three	Agency, identity and personhood in the social sciences	27
four	Frailty	45
five	Understanding abjection	57
six	The moral imperative of care	73
seven	Care work	93
eight	Care without limits	111
nine	Conclusion	127
References		139
Index		173

Preface

As societies across the developed world grow older, the unitary category of old age is dissolving. The growing opportunities offered by what we have called 'third age cultures' clash with the indignities imagined by age's 'other', the fourth age, creating flux out of old certainties (Gilleard and Higgs, 2000; Higgs and Gilleard, 2015). While there is an expanding body of literature on the topic of the third age and its various representations as 'active', 'healthy', 'productive' or 'successful' ageing, the darker elements of later life seem to be obscured rather than revealed in much gerontological writing. But those elements still loom over an ever-extending life course, bunching up especially at its extremes. This book is concerned with this darker imaginary, with age's infirmities, indignities and the ambivalence that lies at the heart of care. These issues pose serious problems for our notions of self-hood and the social ontology of living under the shadow of a fourth age.

The fourth age is, we argue, an idea, a feared imaginary of what old age 'really' is. It is an imaginary that is rooted in the observable experience of frailty and infirmity, of abjection and shame, limited agency and the various social realisations of what we call 'the moral imperative of care'. In this book, we are particularly concerned with examining the nature of personhood and the place of care in both resisting and in realising the fourth age's imaginary. Our aim is to pursue this theoretical framework of the fourth age to help make sense of caring for people in advanced old age. In particular, we wish to explore the Janus-like nature of care, and how its narratives and practices serve sometimes to protect and sometimes to erode social agency, personal identity and human subjectivity. The ambiguity of care is as inescapable as the conditions of frailty and abjection that elicit the fourth age's imaginary. The struggles over agency, identity and subjectivity are present from the beginning to the endings of caring. Rather than assume that such abstractions as 'an ethics of care' or 'an ideology of personhood' can act as reliable guides to secure viable practices of care, we argue that the darkness of the fourth age cannot be separated from the practices and social relations of care. It is necessary, we argue, to recognise that the moral imperative of care is also where the fourth age is realised. At the same time, it represents the social location where that imaginary can best be constrained.

The performances of care have no predetermined end. Their particular realisations are not inherent in the physical constitution of frailty nor in the social nature of abjection, although both are critical in instituting and organising care. Care has its limits, but where and how these are reached is indeterminate, the play of human agents being rarely simple matters of choice. That this is so makes care a concern not only for individuals as persons, but for many of the institutions of our collectively ageing societies. We do not claim to offer a resolution of what is to be done, as we do not believe there is any one resolution for the problems presented by the fourth age. By clarifying some of the underlying narratives and practices of care that serve to embed the social imaginary of 'real' old age within society, we hope at least to offer scope for doing some things differently.

ONE

Old age and the fourth age paradigm

The world's population is ageing at an unprecedented rate. If an 'ageing society' is defined as one where at least 10% of the population is aged 65 years and above, the number of such ageing societies is projected to increase from 59 in 2010 to 138 in 2050 (UN, 2014). By 2050 the world will be home to some 1.5 billion people aged 65 and over, more agedness than the world has ever experienced. Not only are there increasing numbers of ageing societies (Hyde and Higgs, 2016), but some of the already ageing societies are undergoing a process of 'hyper-ageing' as their 65 year old and over populations are projected to increase to over 25% of their respective populations, while the proportion of under 65 year olds falls below average replacement rate fertility (Rowland, 2009). These unprecedented demographic changes have fuelled interest in what has been variously called 'extreme', 'deep' or 'real' old age (Leaf, 1982; Degnen, 2007).

As part of this interest in 'extreme' ageing, the concept of a 'fourth age' has emerged to highlight some of the more unsettling aspects of later life (Higgs and, Gilleard 2015). This concept provides the context for this book, the idea of a feared and impotent old age, and the part that is played by care in realising this imaginary. We begin, in this first chapter, by exploring the various ways that the concept of a fourth age can be understood. Although we focus largely on work carried out since the term was introduced to the literature by Peter Laslett in his seminal work, *A fresh map of life* (Laslett, 1989, 1996), we also examine some of the earlier research that has served as a precursor to contemporary understandings. We then outline our own conceptualisation of the fourth age, as a social imaginary realised within the collective consciousness of society, and set this in contradistinction to other models that see the fourth age located more firmly within the corporeality and/or chronology of individual persons.

As the active, healthy and productive side of ageing has been promoted in the contemporary literature of ageing studies and gerontology, we believe it is now important to balance these accounts of what is often called 'successful ageing' (Rowe and Kahn, 1987) by giving some thought to the darker side of ageing, to the failings of old age and what this might mean for society and for our own future selves. This is not to deny the enormous transformation of later life within today's developed economies and the expansion of what elsewhere we have called the 'cultural field(s) of the third age' (Gilleard and Higgs, 2000, 2005), but as those fields expanded, making later life a larger and more varied space within individual lives and within society, one indirect consequence has been to push the darker side of ageing into the shadows. If the third age can be understood (in part at least) as the cultural expression of successful ageing, the fourth age represents old age as failure. We believe that it is valuable to interrogate this representation, not least so that we can assess how, if at all, we might help ourselves and others to 'fail better'. While some might judge it unwise or even prejudicial to entertain any negative framing of old age, we believe such explorations are now more necessary than ever as the world faces an uncertain future with the emergence of 'hyper-ageing' societies.

Modelling the fourth age

As noted above, the term 'the fourth age' is of relatively recent origin. It remains somewhat controversial in gerontological circles, and has not been the subject of much serious analysis. In order to make a start, it is helpful to map out some of the terrain that appears to prefigure its use, and three models serve as our basic templates. The first derives from demographic considerations, particularly the rise of the 'oldest old' as a proportion of the over-60 population. This model draws on a venerable historical tradition of dividing the life course into stages (Burrow, 1986; Sears, 1986). Within this 'stages of life' framework a distinction has long been made between an earlier 'vital', 'green' or 'mature' old age preceding a later 'decrepit', 'impotent' or 'senile' old age, itself preceding death. Pre-modern accounts of this two stages model of old age have employed a variety of chronological ages in demarcating between them. More modern accounts sought to place the divide around the age of 75, and more recently at 80 or even 85. Neugarten (1974) first referred to this distinction as 'the young old' (aged 55 to 74) in contrast to 'the old old' (aged 75+). Suzman and Riley (1985) later described this older group as 'the oldest old' (aged 85+). The point of all such versions of this model is that the fourth age is assumed to be a stage of life marked by chronology.

The second approach focuses on disability and frailty in later life. Rather than being caught up with chronology and its demographic framing, this model focuses on the distinction between able-bodiedness and infirmity, between the fit and the frail. This approach, too, can be traced back to the categorisation within the Western Christian tradition of those who were unable to fend for themselves by reasons of misfortune rather than as a consequence of their own actions. Along with orphans and widows, the aged sick formed a distinct and deserving class made up of those who were entitled to alms and charity, and later to more formal systems of poor relief. With the dissolution of the Poor Law system in the early 20th century, the newly emerging welfare states attempted to devise a chronological basis for determining relief for old age – in the form of pensions – while employing a 'chronic sickness/disability/infirmity' criterion for determining access to health and social care (Gilleard and Higgs, 2011a). This latter distinction elevated infirmity (frailty, as it is now called) as the point of demarcation around the fourth age, as the aged infirm whose needs for health and social care were based on neither capital nor chronology, but their corporeal weakness. In this second model, frailty and infirmity define the fourth age.

A third model can be discerned, related to, but sufficiently distinct from, the second. It has fewer historical roots, and focuses on proximity to death rather than distance from birth. It is based on the concept of a bio-psychologically distinct phase of life, representing a stage of 'terminal decline'. Advocates of this model have argued for a qualitatively and quantitatively distinct pattern of decline in mental and physical functioning in the final year(s) before death (Kleemeier, 1962; Riegel and Riegel, 1972). Its theoretical formulation has been succinctly summarised by Palmore and Cleveland:

> The essence of this theory is that many human functions are not primarily related to chronological age as such but tend to show marked decline prior to death during a period ranging from a few weeks to a few years. A corollary is that normal aged persons are able to maintain most of their functions on a fairly stable level until they enter the terminal decline phase shortly before death. The theory assumes that whatever combination of genetic and environmental factors causes death also causes the marked decline in functions prior to death. (Palmore and Cleveland, 1976, p 76)

Although the 'theory' of terminal decline was originally formulated in terms of a decline in measured cognitive functioning, more recently it has been extended to cover a much wider range of functions, ranging from motor activity and short-term memory span all the way through to self-perceived health and subjective wellbeing (Gerstorf et al, 2013). Evidence of terminal decline across so many aspects of functioning has led some writers to propose a 'two-stage model' of human ageing, distinguishing between what has been called a 'pre-terminal' phase of relative stability in psychological functioning and a shorter, 'terminal' phase of decline lasting from a few years to as long as a decade prior to death (Bäckman and MacDonald, 2006; Gerstorf and Ram, 2013). While the former has been seen as being subject to secular change, the latter has been considered relatively fixed in its trajectory (Gerstorf et al, 2010).

Although neither Neugarten nor Kleemeier made mention of the term 'the fourth age', their formulations presume an inherent duality to old age – a 'good' versus a 'bad' old age, with 'successful' versus 'unsuccessful' outcomes. This latter distinction – 'successful' versus 'unsuccessful' ageing – has gained considerable traction since it was first outlined by Rowe and Kahn in their paper on 'usual' versus 'successful' ageing. They intended to challenge what they called 'a gerontology of the usual' by stressing the distinction between normal ageing as disease-free healthy ageing and 'ageing as usual', with its accompanying 'natural' decline (Rowe and Kahn, 1987, p 143). Subsequent use of the term has, however, tended to elide 'usual' with 'successful', such that ageing is increasingly represented as usual and successful, with pathological or unsuccessful ageing treated as the exception to this rule (Strawbridge et al, 2002). Given this confounding of normal and usual, it is unsurprising that studies examining the prevalence of 'successful' ageing have produced widely differing views of its 'normality', from a low of 0.4% to a high of 95.0% (Depp and Jeste, 2006).

What constitutes the antithesis of 'successful ageing'? For Rowe and Kahn it was 'normal' or 'usual' ageing, but little by little an alternative and somewhat darker picture has prevailed – that of failed age and frail old people. While Kahn acknowledged that those not designated successful risked being judged 'unsuccessful and therefore as failing', he considered such binary thinking more a question of an American 'succeed-or-fail' world view than any necessary consequence of the concept of successful ageing (Kahn, 2002, p 726). Others have been less sure, arguing that successful ageing models:

> ... have been and continue to be criticized for being most applicable to the relatively healthy "third age" of life or "young old" populations and not to the "fourth age" or the "oldest old" which comes with significant constraints in functional capacity, frailty and psychological losses, and

> limited effectiveness of interventions. (Flatt et al, 2013, p 947)

The term itself – 'the fourth age' – can be traced back to Peter Laslett's book, *A new map of life*. Laslett, however, was not really concerned with 'deep' old age. His main aim was to articulate an alternative, more aspirational view of later life, based on his concept of a 'third age' (Laslett, 1989, 1996). For Laslett, the concept of a fourth age merely provided a sharp contrast to the third. At the same time, in his new map of the life course, the fourth age follows the third in a transition that he describes as 'greater than either of the previous life course transitions'. As a period 'of dependence and decrepitude' (Laslett, 1996, pp 192-4), the fourth age marks 'the onset of final decline' when people become merely 'passengers or encumbrances' (Laslett, 1996, p 194). By promoting the opportunities of a successful third age, Laslett, like Rowe and Kahn, ended up inadvertently focusing on the failures of the fourth age. The only positive suggestion Laslett offered as regards this stage of life was that future generations of third agers might develop the wisdom better to manage the transition, or preferably, learn how to put it off for as long as possible, thereby limiting its presence and significance within the life course.

A different approach has been followed by Paul Baltes, who cut his research teeth modelling patterns of intellectual change over the life course when he became a powerful critic of the assumption of universal decline in mental and behavioural competence in later life (Baltes and Schaie, 1978; Baltes, 1987; Baltes and Baltes, 1990). In his later work, he began to question the limits to the plasticity of mental and behavioural competence. Adopting an explicit 'stages of life' approach, he wrote:

> For the younger-old, those in the Third Age, the prospects seem bright ... modern societies have the potential to create a better future for the younger of the older ages and ... empower individuals to become "successful agers" [but] for most of the older-old however the prospects are not so bright. From my point of view "hope with a mourning band" may be the motto best suited to this situation.... As demographers celebrate each month gained in the lives of the oldest-old, researchers focused on improving quality of life worry about the associated increase in the gap between longevity and vitality. (Baltes, 2006, p 38)

For Baltes and Smith (1999, 2003) there exists a fundamental difference in the capacities and adaptability of people before and after the age of 80. They represent this difference as an increased dependency on culture and society concomitant with a reduced capacity to benefit or learn from these external sources. At this stage of life, risk of adverse outcomes multiplies while the capacity to overcome disease, dysfunction and external stress is radically diminished.

In formulating this model, Baltes was drawing on a chronologically bound 'stages of life' model that presumes qualitative as well as quantitative differences between one period of later life and another. At the same time he uses a variant of the terminal decline model to define those differences. Like Laslett, he drew on the idea of a final decline whose trajectory is unlikely to be halted, let alone reversed, and which involves decline across multiple domains. In that sense, this imputed final decline is distinct from the development of chronic or degenerative disease, whether it is cancer, dementia or heart disease, which initially at least represent deleterious processes within discrete organ systems in the absence of other diseases or dysfunctions. In this sense the Baltes model approaches and overlaps with Fried's model of frailty that treats frailty as an age-related syndrome of multi-system failure, separate from disease and disability, and which leads toward 'an end stage' that is 'irreversible and presage[s] death' (Fried et al, 2001, M154). This link between frailty and the fourth age is explored in some detail later in the book.

Social imaginary of a fourth age

While Neugarten and Riley wanted to break up the 'indeterminate' length of old age into chronological segments, Laslett (and, to some extent, Baltes) sought to frame the fourth age as a more distinctly definitive stage of life, that of 'late' later life. Others have pursued the idea that a qualitative change takes place in later life, much as Baltes has argued, but one that is linked not with years lived but with proximity to death. In order to avoid the impossibility of determining this 'terminal stage' during life, formulations have been made that represent this 'terminal stage' as a state of 'multi-system deterioration' that anticipates or prefigures a steep and seemingly irreversible pathway toward ever more adverse outcomes leading to death – what might be called the 'frailing of old age' (Gilleard and Higgs, 2011a).

We have proposed an alternative view of the fourth age that seeks to understand it as a cultural or social imaginary, framed by humanity's collective experience of decline and deterioration in later life (Gilleard and Higgs, 2013). In thinking about the fourth age like this, we have drawn an analogy with a phenomenon from astrophysics, treating the fourth age as a 'black hole' about whose nature we can only speculate, restricting any attempts at measurement or understanding to observing not the phenomenon itself, but disturbances around its 'event horizon' (Gilleard and Higgs, 2010).

In this sense our model of the fourth age is one that functions as a social or cultural imaginary, fashioned more by the meanings we attribute to old age than by any set of biological or psychological indicators. These meanings have both historical roots and contemporary resonance. Their roots are reflected in old distinctions between seniority and senility, between the sturdy and the infirm, between a ripe and a rotten old age. By contrast, contemporary influences mirror the growing cultural significance of the third age, of new ageing lifestyles as well as a late life consumerist habitus that suggests that through the 'consumption' of various products and practices, individuals can remain more or less active participants in third age lifestyles until they choose to drop out or die. Beside the 'drivers' of choice, autonomy, self-expression and pleasure associated with third age culture lies a fear of an unacceptable ageing. Ageing without agency, free-falling into a deep and uncomfortable old age is what frames the kind of old age that the cultures of the third age seem to mask or repress (Gilleard and Higgs, 2010; Higgs and Gilleard, 2015).

The notion that there is a 'real' old age, waiting to emerge from beneath the surface of 'normal' or 'usual' old age, one that incorporates all the negative aspects of late life, is not an academic conceit. Its social expression has been brought into sharp focus by a study of ageing in a small community reported by Degnen (2007). She refers to the

> ... distinctions made by older people themselves about the boundaries and distinctions between "real" and "normal" old age. While a great deal of physical change and a certain amount of shifts in mental states are accommodated in older people's views of normal ageing, the most important gauge of the onset of real old age is a decline in mental acuity and related shifts in comportment. (Degnen, 2007, p 79)

Degnen highlights the active construction of the idea of a 'real' old age by older people themselves, arising from observations made within and between their age peers. Such distinctions, she suggests, are more acutely observed by older people themselves than by those not yet old, who are not yet participants in 'third age' cultures, and for whom such boundaries and distinctions have yet to attain any 'real' personal significance.

Our view of the fourth age is that it serves as an imagined boundary within later life, a divide created in part by age peers, by professionals and by public opinion. It embodies something more disturbing and more threatening than the mere weight of chronology, something darker than disease or disability. As an imaginary, it is not new. It is not itself the product of 'modern' life but draws on a long cultural history of distinguishing between the good and the bad sides of later life. As the cultures of the third age, of ageing 'successfully', have come so much to the fore in recent times, these other aspects of 'real' old age have acquired a deeper, darker and more marginal existence as they are pushed from centre stage by the opportunities and optimism highlighted by an expanding third age culture. It is all the more timely, then, to take another, closer and more considered look at the various elements that make up this imaginary, in order better to outline the nature of its 'disturbances' within the field of later life.

Elements of the fourth age imaginary

Four elements underpin much of the social imaginary of the fourth age – frailty, abjection, the loss of agency and care (Higgs and Gilleard, 2015). We treat frailty here as the equivalent of infirmity, in the sense of how the 'aged and infirm' were once singled out, along with orphans and widows, 'the halt and the lame', 'the blind, the deaf and the dumb', as co-constituents in the broad category of the 'deserving poor' rather than in any 'technical' or 'biomedical' sense (Gilleard and Higgs 2011a). Thus conceived, frailty encompasses both mental and physical infirmity, and implies both a material and a moral vulnerability. The frail are necessarily 'at risk' in the environment and in the community. We explore frailty further in Chapter 4. The second element or component of the fourth age is abjection. By abjection, we mean all those aspects of infirmity that society finds most distasteful – the fourth age's material and moral repugnance. The abjection of the fourth age carries different connotations. It reflects in part of a social location, a category of person or an abject class. But even more so, it represents the inability to look after oneself that is deepened by the inability to acknowledge one's own inabilities. This inability to share in the construction of one's inabilities as well as an inability to assert oneself as a potential agent means, in effect, that the individual fails to be the subject of their own inabilities. Abjection is further discussed in Chapter 5.

The combination of frailty and abjection implies a moral responsibility for others to care for those to whom such frailty and abjection are attributed. This moral responsibility is not unique to the fourth age. It has long been shared with the needs of other deserving groups whose vulnerabilities have been acknowledged in the provision made for widows and orphans and other categories of the 'impotent poor'. The moral imperative of care, as well as the various narratives and practices of care underpinned by it, are addressed in the final three chapters of this book. In these chapters we examine the central paradox whereby care both shapes and is shaped by the social imaginary of the fourth age. Whether provided informally by family and friends, or formally by public or private institutions, care is both a response to, and a definer of, needs; it involves narratives and practices that can work together or that can lead to conflicts and contradictions. Care evokes complex feelings and judgements in and about the person being cared for and the person doing the caring. In the circumstances of advanced old age, care is carried out under the shadow of the fourth age, and often continues through its deepest shadows, at the end of life.

Agency and the loss of agency make up the fourth component framing the fourth age's social imaginary. In many ways the concepts of agency, identity and personhood pose the most difficult problems, reflecting some of the more intractable preoccupations of modern thought, in philosophy and in medicine as well as in the behavioural and social sciences. These are central issues in this book because they are critical to care and the management and organisation of care in advanced old age. In the chapters that immediately follow this introduction, we outline some of the ways that these terms have been understood, in philosophy and in the social and behavioural sciences, before considering how they have been employed in formulating models of care and standards of professional practice in helping mentally and physically frail older people. We hope that this helps set the context for a more engaged consideration of care under the shadows of the fourth age.

Conclusions

This book addresses the question of care and personhood in the fourth age. While the fourth age can be thought of as a stage of life or as a condition of infirmity in later life, we have chosen to frame it as a 'social imaginary'. By this we mean that the fourth age crystallises the collective interpretations of all that is most feared about old age, its impotence and infirmity, its indignity and the dependency that seems to surround the social position of those at the extremes of later life. Whatever may be the subjective experiences of individual infirm older people, this collective imaginary creates or sustains a set of assumptions and attributions that impel others to seek to care for those assigned to the fourth age at the same time as invoking a degree of ambivalence towards those being cared for.

The fourth age imaginary reflects society's interpretations of late life frailty, its abjection and helplessness and the need for care that accompanies evident dependency. Accompanying such interpretations of frailty and need is a sense of difference, of otherness. For those who are not frail, infirmity and its accompanying abjection make of the old and frail something or rather someone other, and not just other, but something less than themselves. This 'lessness' and 'otherness' that interpellate judgements of agedness and frailty and the need for care bring down, in the very process of realising that care, the shadows of the fourth age just as they purport to hold them at bay. Our aim is to examine and interrogate the complex processes that contribute to care, and the ambivalence realised within the social relationships of care, in the hope that such examination may cast light on what we have called the fourth age, at the risk of an incomplete resolution to the dilemmas posed by the fourth age.

TWO

Interrogating personhood

The fourth age imaginary embodies fears of dependency, frailty and the gradual loss of our sense of agency, identity and our status as persons. This fear, particularly as it is represented in the fear of 'losing one's mind' or of developing Alzheimer's, brings to the fore questions of agency, identity and personhood. When we first wrote about the fourth age, we described it as 'ageing without agency' (Gilleard and Higgs, 2010), treating mental decline as a decline in 'agency'. By so doing we wanted to acknowledge how closely allied fears are of an unwanted old age with fears of losing our mind. The problem of declining mental powers, particularly as represented by dementia or 'senility', is not new, even if it is now represented by the medical terminology of 'Alzheimer's disease and related disorders'. Within this clinical discourse, Alzheimer's was described by some clinicians as causing, or constituting, 'a loss of self' or even a 'social death' (Sweeting and Gilhooly, 1997; Cohen and Eisdorfer, 2001). In this and the following chapter we interrogate the term 'personhood' and its status, whether in shaping or resisting the fourth age's social imaginary.

Personhood has been used with increasing frequency in the academic, clinical and professional literature on the care of infirm, especially mentally infirm, old people. Acknowledging the personhood of people with dementia has become one of the defining aspects of contemporary policy and practice in this field (Jenkins and Price, 1996; NICE, 2006; Dewing, 2008; Nuffield Council on Bioethics, 2009; Thomas and Milligan, 2015). Personhood is invoked, for example, as the basis for 'person-centred' care in institutional settings and in the instigation of calls for a 'politics of citizenship' for people diagnosed with dementia (McCormack, 2001; Bartlett and O'Connor 2010). The work of Tom Kitwood in particular has been a touchstone for many of those grappling with the issue of personhood and dementia (Baldwin and Capstick, 2007).In a number of works, Kitwood outlined what he saw as the fundamental denial of personhood in care settings for people with dementia (Kitwood, 1993, 1997a; Kitwood and Bredin, 1992). Under the influence of the extreme individualism that has dominated Western societies, personhood, he claimed, has been reduced to two criteria: autonomy and rationality (Kitwood, 1997a, p 9). This reduction of the term to such an individualised notion of 'cognitive competence' has profound implications for the moral recognition of people with mental impairments, whether acquired later in life or as problems of childhood development. As a counter to this, Kitwood contended that personhood should be conceptualised differently, so that relationships and moral solidarity become its foundational principles, in order to overcome the 'social psychology that is malignant in its effects' (Kitwood, 1997a, p 14).

While much of value has since been written on the importance of maintaining personhood in the care of people with dementia (Innes et al, 2004; McCormack, 2004), we would argue that Kitwood and other advocates of person-centred care for dementia have failed adequately to explore the meanings that can be attached to personhood. As a result, the term has been used mostly as a signifier of 'good' care and its absence indicative of 'bad' care. Since care rarely has any completely satisfying conclusion, it is difficult to know whether or not the deployment of 'personhood' has played a central role in improving care. In this and the following chapter, we examine the issue of personhood in the wider literature of philosophy and its applicability to dementia care, as well as to the care of infirm older people more generally. In so doing we provide an explicit critique of Kitwood's position and how it renders problematic those narratives of care that are derived, in whole or in part, from it. We outline how thinking about personhood depends on ideas of self, personal identity, agency and consciousness. While each of these concepts can be seen as constitutive of personhood, each has been thought of differently. These differences in ways of understanding the constituents of personhood result in various possible versions of personhood. This has led some writers to conclude that the status of personhood is 'logically confused and morally objectionable' (Sapontzis, 1981, p 607). Such difficulties in employing personhood in any consistent and coherent manner consequently make its status both for understanding dementia and for orientating the narratives and practices of care problematic, and maybe ultimately best avoided.

In interrogating ideas about personhood we also seek to explore its extension to debates concerning the 'dividing practices' that separate a third from a fourth age in later life (Grenier, 2007; Higgs and Gilleard, 2015). We do this not to undermine the motivations lying behind person-centred care, nor the advocacy of the rights of individuals with dementia, but rather to avoid expanding what appears to be an increasing gap between the professionalised rhetoric of care and its everyday social realities. We argue that the danger of placing such a slippery concept as personhood at the centre of any set of organisational practices of care risks undermining rather than enhancing the fundamental moral imperative of care that we believe is central to the social realities of a disabled and disabling old age. The major purpose of this chapter is to justify such a call for caution by deconstructing the debates within philosophy around the identity of persons and personhood. In Chapter 3 we turn to more sociologically informed discussions in order to identify points for a more pragmatic approach to the care of older persons.

The ambivalence of 'persons'

In response to what he considered the lack of any theory guiding the care of people with dementia, Kitwood chose to make personhood central to his theory (Kitwood and Bredin, 1992, p 270). At first, he made little reference to others' theories of personhood, satisfying himself with the view that personhood was not so much given as 'acquired' during development as a result of relationships with others. This development was presaged on the relationship between an infant and its mother/caregiver, and later extended to incorporate other relationships (Kitwood and Bredin, 1992, p 276). Being or becoming a person, in turn, gives an individual a unique moral status, making him or her worthy of moral respect (Kitwood and Bredin, 1992, p 275). Later, Kitwood makes more reference to others' ideas, particularly the work of philosopher and theologian Martin Buber and his concept of a person as a 'thou' rather than a 'you'. By this, he means, in Buber's terms, relating to someone as a 'pure being', without instrumentality or other ulterior purpose (Kitwood, 1997b, pp 5-6). Personhood is presented not as an empirically verifiable concept, but as a statement of moral fact. A person is a 'thou', and recognising another's being as a 'thou' is the essence of making that person a person.

The term 'personhood' already had considerable use in philosophy well before Buber employed the term, and it continues to be a topic of philosophical debate. Although the history is complicated, it is fair to say that its explication has been within either 'moral' or 'metaphysical' traditions (Beauchamp, 1999, p 309). Both traditions provide responses to the question 'what is a person?', and both address issues of identity and, by implication, self-hood. While attempts to establish the nature of self and personal identity are largely the domain of metaphysics, moral philosophy has been more concerned with the moral identity or status of persons. In so far as dementia has been a subject of interest to psychiatry, psychology and the neurosciences, it is unsurprising that these disciplines have all drawn on the metaphysics of personhood (Hughes et al, 2006; Hughes, 2013). Based on its use as 'a foundational concept in many systems of ethics', it is equally unsurprising that law, medicine and theology have been more closely involved with moral considerations of personhood (Dworkin, 1993; Dresser, 1995; Jaworska, 1999; Post, 2006; Kittay and Carlson 2010).

As we go on to show, defining personhood within metaphysics has led, in turn, to debates about its constituent parts – agency, identity, reflexivity and will. Debates within moral philosophy have been about the moral status of personhood, and whether or not it is anything more than a 'placeholder' for claiming rights. In both cases, the question remains what added value the term possesses either over its constituent parts (in the case of metaphysics) or over the status of simply being human (in the case of moral philosophy and human rights). The difficulty in both cases of finding the term's unique selling point suggests that it may be covering up more than it reveals.

Personhood as metaphysical identity

'Identity' and 'self' are closely related concepts that have long been at the heart of what has been known as metaphysics, that branch of philosophy concerned with the questions of ontology, the nature of being and existence. In reviewing the sources of the self within the Western intellectual tradition, Charles Taylor has made the point that articulating a distinction between an inner 'me' and an outer world made up of things that are 'not me' constitutes 'a historically limited mode of self-interpretation ... dominant in the modern West' (Taylor, 1992, p 111). Many other writers have also traced the modern Western tradition back to René Descartes, who is generally seen to be the first thinker to make the distinction between knowledge gained from within – the *cogito* – and knowledge gained from without – the material world and its quasi mechanical workings (Taylor, 1992, p 156). Once this distinction was made it raised the further question of whether or not it is possible to comprehend the nature of self and personal identity without having to resort to external knowledge based on the material body. One solution was to treat 'self' and 'personhood' as entities that could not be reduced to, or assimilated within, the category of material bodies. Instead, such capacities were seen as existing in a contingent relationship with the body, a relationship that Strawson has claimed was irreducible to what he called basic or primary particulars – namely, matter (Strawson, 1971). As a consequence of this, if the self and personal identity can be seen as the constituents of 'persons', one way of determining who or what a 'person' is, is to establish whether or not he or she is capable of 'owning' a state of consciousness. Although states of consciousness may vary in time and form, what provides them with any unity is their being necessarily 'a person's' consciousness and not just a thing sufficient in and of itself.

Another doyen of the Enlightenment, John Locke, began his *Essay concerning human understanding* by expressing a similar intention to that of Descartes, namely, of wanting to start thinking about the self or subject free of any preconceptions. Locke wanted to establish a new and more objective understanding of humanity based on the consciousness of a distinct self that he saw as the hallmark of a person. Personal identity existed because of consciousness, or rather it existed because of that aspect of consciousness that identifies itself with all previous actions and experiences 'in what bodies soever they appear or what substances soever that consciousness adheres to' (Locke, 1975, p 347). For Locke, not identity but consciousness of one's identity was all defining. This position was challenged by another Enlightenment thinker, David Hume. Hume pointed out that because all consciously entertained ideas, impressions and perceptions are essentially fleeting, consciousness is not continuous but fragmentary, and hence the conscious self must also be equally fragmentary. What gave conscious thoughts and experiences their sense of continuity and underlying unity was the faculty of memory. Memory served as the unifier of what otherwise would be a fragmentary self (or selves). Had we no memory, Hume speculated, we would have no means of tying together one impression with another, no sense of causality, no knowledge of 'that chain of causes and effects which constitute our self or person' (Hume, 1978, p 261).

After Hume, philosophical enquiry into the identity of persons went into a kind of abeyance. Instead, the term was employed, most notably by Immanuel Kant, not as a metaphysical conundrum of the self or *cogito*, but as a necessary status for establishing an ethics. Kant can be considered the modern forerunner of the idea of personhood as status, in contradistinction to philosophers such as Locke and Hume who framed it in terms of personal identity. Kant's conception of a person refers to a universal abstract property that renders human beings 'ends' in themselves and thus deserving of respect. He treats as irrelevant biographical as well as biological elements of personal distinctiveness in favour of what Radin has called 'bare abstract rational agents' (Radin, 1982, p 967). While such a position avoids any truck with a metaphysics of the person, it is important as a precursor of viewing personhood in terms not of identity but of its associated rights claims, a theme we return to in a later section.

Turning to present-day writings, echoes of Hume's position can be found in contemporary theories of the self and personhood that represent the self as a fundamentally 'discursive' narrative. In his book *Oneself as another*, Paul Ricoeur distinguished between two aspects of personal identity – sameness (*idem*) and self-hood (*ipse*) (Ricoeur, 1992, p 116). Identity as sameness can be seen as the property of substances – whether human beings or items of clothing. Identity as selfhood does not work in this way. As Ricoeur puts it, selfhood is a question of who, not what, we are, while character (or personality), he suggests, lies somewhere between the two, such that the stability or sameness of character elides 'who I am' with 'what I am'. Selfhood is unequivocally about the former. For Ricoeur, self-hood (who I am) is hence a matter of 'narrative identity' – what Alistair MacIntyre termed 'the narrative unity of a life' (quoted in Ricoeur, 1992, p 158). This narrative unity, Ricoeur claims, enables narrative identity to link two aspects of sameness or identity with one another, 'the permanence in time of character and that of self-constancy' (Ricoeur, 1992, p 166).

Persons and selves

Ricoeur treats the self as the central part of our identity as persons, alongside our sameness as both matter and character. In that sense, the term 'person' – or personal identity – includes the idea of self and 'other'. Although both Locke and Hume had treated the person as more or less equivalent to the self, some contemporary philosophers have tended to distinguish between them. Remaining the same 'person' is not considered equivalent to retaining the same 'self'. Even if, as Schechtman (1994) has put it, 'person-identity' and 'self-identity' should be co-extensive, 'for a richer and fuller life', such co-extensivity is neither theoretically nor empirically necessary. Selves can remain the same selves even if they are no longer the same persons (and presumably, vice versa).

Is a degree of co-extensivity between personal identity and self-identity required as a criterion of 'personhood' in the same way that a degree of psychological continuity is required for personal identity to persist in time? Parfit argues that there are so many obstacles to determining whether or not human beings retain a continuous personal identity that it is more useful to consider this as a matter of degree rather than as a matter of categorical presence or absence (Parfit, 1984). For Parfit, there are always degrees of psychological continuity in individuals' lives, some more, some less, and some less in some periods of our lives while more in other periods. Personal identity and self-hood are, he argues, better thought of not as singular entities at all, but rather as matters of degree, such that we are sometimes more and sometimes less 'ourselves', a self that is always subject to what Ricoeur calls degrees of 'narrative unity'.

There are, nevertheless, 'limit conditions' to this unity of the self, such that, as Schechtman has put it, 'radical enough psychological change literally brings about a loss of identity' (Schechtman, 2003, p 242). One element of such 'limit conditions' is the rate of change or of loss – with slower rates of change representing greater possibilities for maintaining continuity in the face of change in contrast to rapid and violent change. She refers to a second limitation in maintaining sufficient self-sameness (or the unity of the self) as narrative coherence – the extent to which the individual can maintain a coherent story of continuing to be the 'I' he or she always was, despite marked or even sudden changes to life, self and circumstance.

Even if these considerations capture some of the conditions necessary for or inimical to sustaining psychological continuity, 'they are', she argues, still 'missing a piece and this piece ... is empathic access' (Schechtman, 2003, p 245). She defines empathic access as when a person 'retains some sympathy for the psychological features of the life phase to which she retains access' (Schechtman, 2003, p 255); in other words, so long as an individual retains some memory of past phases or periods in their life, and those memories include 'feeling part of' that memory, then no matter what disjunctures or losses occur, the bond of 'warm memory' preserves psychological continuity – and thereby our survival as selves. What is important for Schechtman is the empathic access, the anticipation of loss and the disconnection from the selves and others that peopled our past. Perhaps, as Parfit claims, our survival – as persons or as selves – is not so important after all. What matters are the processes that constitute our survival, those of managing change, maintaining coherence and retaining affective memories (Parfit, 2003a). Perhaps it matters less whether or not we retain a sense of identity as 'sameness' so long as we retain these empathic qualities of personhood to which Schechtman has referred – of feeling 'attached' to our past and our present (Schechtman, 2003).

Persons as agents

So far our attention has been on consciousness as experience – of memory and feelings, the sense of being oneself. But, as Korsgaard has pointed out, 'a person is both active and passive, both an agent and a subject of experiences' (Korsgaard, 1989, p 101). In the 1970s

Harry Frankfurt questioned formulations of personhood that relied simply on some combination of possessing a particular human body and possessing consciousness (Frankfurt, 1971). He argued that 'one essential difference between persons and other creatures is to be found in the structure of a person's will' (Frankfurt, 1971, p 6). Frankfurt made the distinction between the presence of desires and motives and the capacity to make choices and what he called 'second-order desires', desires to be more or less what one is, desires to be and to act differently. He distinguished between persons with 'volitions of the second order' and individuals who, although possessing rationality, have no such second-order volitions, no desires to be other than how they are or how they act. These latter he calls 'wantons', humans but not quite persons. Korsgaard likewise argues that what determines personhood or personal identity (Ricoeur's *'ipse'*) is not the absence of change in our appearance, attitudes, habits or way of life, but the authorship of change (Korsgaard, 1989, p 123). Authorship, of course, has resonance with Ricoeur's idea of the narrative unity of the self; however, what Frankfurt and Korsgaard focus on is not so much narrative but performative agency.

Daniel Dennett has drawn on Frankfurt's notion of second-order volition in outlining those criteria that he believed must be met in order for individuals to possess 'personhood' (Dennett, 1976). To have the status of 'personhood', he argued, an individual must be capable of having second-order intentions, as well as possessing rationality, must be able to be judged conscious, must be treated by others as if the individual is a person, must be capable of reciprocating others' feelings, beliefs and attitudes, must be able to communicate with others and must be capable of self-consciousness. For Dennett as for others, neither continuity over time nor identity with past selves is required. His formulation of personhood stresses not identity per se but rather the capacities or qualities that an individual possesses at any one point in time. The definition is also not contingent on whether or not these qualities persist. Thus, one may acquire personhood without always having had it, and by implication one can lose personhood despite once having had it, depending on the degree of retention or loss of each of these capacities or qualities.

Other attempts have been made to define the relationship between persons and agency drawing on similar ideas to those outlined by Frankfurt and Dennett. Charles Taylor has raised the question in the following way: 'What do we mean by a person? Certainly an agent, with purposes, desires, aversions and so forth. But obviously more than this because many animals can be considered agents in this sense, but we don't consider them persons' (Taylor, 1985, p 237). Following from this, Taylor treats agency as an illustration of Frankfurt's first-order volitions or Dennett's intentional systems. He then adds: 'we conceive of [a person] as a special kind of agent, an agent-plus, who can also make life plans, hold values, choose' (Taylor, 1985, p 261) as well as being 'an agent who has an understanding of self as an agent' (Taylor, 1985, p 263). Here he is including Dennett's criteria of reflexivity informing actions. Finally, he states: 'it is not just that we are aware of ourselves as agents ... [but] we also have a sense of certain standards which apply to us as self-aware agents' (Taylor, 1985, p 263). In short, persons are not just agents, they are not just reflexive or second-order agents; rather, they are moral agents capable of experiencing guilt and shame. Agency is a necessary but insufficient aspect of being a person, a self; even metaphysical agency is insufficient. For Taylor, moral agency is demanded. By substituting 'moral agency' for 'metaphysical agency' Taylor distinguishes between the initiation and planning of behaviour or actions from the planning of behaviour against a set of internal criteria that can be articulated before and after the action, an agency that is attached to moral narratives. This distinction between types or levels of agency is important. Human beings – persons – are not just capable of choosing or wanting to do something; they are capable of wanting to do other than they do, of wanting to be other than they are. In short, for Taylor as for Frankfurt, they are capable of second-order desires. The difference is that Taylor calls this moral agency.

Personhood and moral status

Dennett, perhaps more clearly than Taylor, has differentiated between metaphysical and moral notions of a 'person'. To transform personhood into moral personhood, he states, an extra dimension of 'accountability' needs to be added. He gives as an example of this distinction the position of an insane man who is not treated in law as accountable but with whom other, non-insane persons interact in ways otherwise 'indistinguishable from normal personal relations' (Dennett, 1976, p 177). 'Accountability' is not required for 'basic' (metaphysical) personhood, but is required for 'moral' personhood. This notion of moral personhood as a 'higher' order of personhood than mere 'metaphysical' personhood reflects the importance given to agency over identity in such formulations. How far, then, do moral agency, moral identity and moral status converge in thinking about personhood within an ethical or moral philosophical tradition? While metaphysics has pursued the relationship between agency, identity and personhood (or selfhood), these inquiries subsume two distinct motives. One, a relatively neutral line of questioning, asks what confers unity to ourselves – how and to what extent we develop and retain a sense of personal identity, of being the person we are – in short, exploring the constituents of personhood and our sense of self. The other, less neutral and of more social than personal concern, is what distinguishes persons from other sentient beings – what makes individuals 'human' and what consequences should follow from that. While the search for the necessary criteria of personhood may seem on the surface a metaphysical inquiry, a reflection of human curiosity, a search to know ourselves 'from the inside', inseparable from such inquiries, is a concern with status or standing, and by implication the grading of persons. It is to this question that we now turn. It is more a question of moral status than any metaphysics of personhood, and arguably it is these issues of moral status that underlie Kitwood's account of personhood and person-centred care much more than any concern with the metaphysics of personal identity.

Although, as we noted earlier, Kant's abstract concept of personhood provides one of the foundations for realising the moral identity of persons as ends in themselves, the clearest statement concerning the link between personhood rights and status comes from the idealist philosopher Hegel, who outlined the imperative to 'be a person and respect others as persons' (Hegel, 1991, p 35). For Hegel, all such rights are personal and, following Kant, derive from the abstract rationality possessed by every human being. Given the universality of personhood as a rights-holding status it cannot be further qualified by any individual, physical or social particularities. But behind that abstract 'species being' lie some unexamined assumptions that suggest a degree of grading in the moral standing of persons.

As Perring has pointed out in relation to access to healthcare: '[most] approaches deciding who deserves treatment and what are the rights of the patient implicitly assume the notion of "degrees of personhood"' (Perring, 1997, p 193). Replacing metaphysical with moral personhood does not avoid having to confront such issues; indeed, it could be argued that it sharpens the confrontation. Any conceptualisation of personhood – whether as a metaphysical or a moral category – that treats it as a matter of degree inhibits the automatic application of any set of rights that are granted on the basis of assuming an 'all or nothing' quality to personhood. If personhood is a matter of degree, the rights that an individual can claim must also be matters of degree, and thereby subject at the very least to some kind of negotiation. In a sense contemporary philosophy can be said to have abandoned the attempt to define a stable continuous self, and has instead opted for a status model of personhood. But, as in the consideration of any other status, this, too, is contingent, relational and normative – in short, a matter of degree.

For some ethicists, this conclusion poses such serious problems that they would prefer to abandon the term altogether, arguing that 'instead of encouraging the development of morality as an all-pervasive fundamental world outlook, it justifies restricting moral concern to the observance of a small number of rules' (Sapontzis, 1981, p 618). For others, reducing the concept of moral personhood to that of a purely normative concept means that 'the ascription of personhood is nothing but our declaration that an entity is a valid object of our moral concern' (Ohlin, 2005, p 237). If so, then establishing the basis for that moral concern and for the application of human rights must lie elsewhere, and cannot reside in the concept of personhood itself.

This presents a key problem that has been addressed by Ohlin, namely, whether or not the concept of the person is a necessary requirement for all human rights claims (Ohlin, 2005). Ohlin notes how legal systems have placed personhood at the centre of human rights. He asks whether it is necessary to prove that a person is indeed a person in order to grant him or her rights. In practice, he suggests personhood serves merely as a 'place marker', treating those who have rights as persons and those who do not as non-persons. In what Parfit (2003b) has called the argument from below, Ohlin argues that it is the necessary constituents of personhood, such as possessing consciousness, and not personhood itself, which determine moral status and in turn confer rights. No additional value is conferred by the status of being a person: its constituents have already done the work. Whether treated as a metaphysical compound or a moral status, Ohlin argues, evacuated of its underpinnings, personhood is essentially a vacuous term.

In their review of the potential neuro-scientific bases for 'personhood', Farah and Heberlein similarly concluded that since it is impossible empirically to defend any specific criteria for personhood, 'rather than ask whether someone or something is a person, we should ask how much capacity exists for enjoying [such qualities as] intelligence, self-awareness, etc' (Farah and Heberlein, 2007, p 46). Yet, as these authors note, the personhood narrative still persists. They sought to resolve this persistent conundrum by claiming that personhood is, in fact, a functional illusion that reflects the way human brains process information about other human beings, a term that cannot be eradicated by intellectual debate because it reflects an evolutionarily determined piece of human neurological hardware.

Whether or not this is the case, personhood has a powerful presence in society, and particularly within most modern legal systems. It is not easy simply to dismiss the term outright, or even replace it with more elemental terms such as 'rationality', 'judgement' or 'autonomy'. Instead, it might be more straightforward to demand one's rights as of right, as a person – what Kant might term as a rights-holder (Kant, 1895) – rather than endlessly seeking to dissect or demonstrate its qualities in any particular instance. In short, personhood may serve to represent the moral identity possessed by each and every human being. This, of course, leads to the question of how, then, to understand not personhood, but that which it serves – namely, the idea of possessing moral identity.

The developmental nature of personhood and its moral identity

Although personhood remains a stubbornly persistent concept, it is not necessary to assume that it is an inherent and unchanging feature of human nature. A more graduated perspective can be found in developmental studies of personhood and self. Thus some philosophers and psychologists have argued that the sense of self emerges and develops through a process of emergent 'second-order' systems of control that become increasingly effective in governing the individual's actions, desires, wants and wishes rather than their being present from the start, in the form of some unchanged and unchanging essence. Such a perspective is evident, for example, in Walter Mischel's operationalisation of the concept of the 'delay of gratification' in the development of a robust agentic self (Mischel, 1974), in Piaget's concept of human development as the process of replacing a limited and limiting set of biological capabilities by a range of successively higher-order capabilities acquired during the course of development (Piaget, 1976), and in Vygotsky's concept of the evolution and internalisation of 'secondary' higher-order thinking through the social media of language and tool use (Vygotsky, 1978). A more general articulation of this point is made by Beauchamp when he argues that we first become human, then human selves, and finally acquire by degrees the status of personhood, eventually learning to exercise 'genuine' agency – in the sense of having volitional control over our desires (Beauchamp, 1999).

Such 'developmentalist' notions can be seen as reflecting the emergence of what Taylor has called 'agency-plus' (Taylor, 1985). The kind of developmental sequence posited above also, however, implies the possibility of an equivalent decline in the capacity for or expression of such 'agency-plus'. If agency and self-hood are matters both of degree and of development, so, too, it would seem must be true of personhood. If personhood is a matter of human development, is it not also subject to human ageing and decline? As metaphysical concerns turn into moral ones, the developmentalist approach becomes more salient and more problematic. While metaphysicians of personal identity have considered questions of sameness arising from ageing, the general consensus has been that changes brought about slowly and imperceptibly, such as those occurring as a consequence of ageing, do not pose any major threat to the identity of persons. The self, it is assumed, maintains its self-same identity through memory and narrative, including its narratives of growing up and growing old. But if personhood is thought of as an acquired status, constituted by increasing reflexivity, higher-order thinking and 'agency-plus', and if these, in turn, serve as precursors of moral standing, then the consequences of this developmentalist approach take on more importance, particularly in the case of age-associated cognitive decline.

Most people would accept, for example, that new-born infants are neither capable of explicit memory nor of reflexivity, and hence would seem not to have acquired status as moral agents. But does their lack of sufficient degrees of personhood have any bearing on their moral standing – as the object of others' care and concern? If personhood and moral agency are acquired, the self or personal identity of the child remains contiguous, and so the acquisition of new qualities and capacities adds to but does not render unidentifiable the self of earlier times. A similar argument can be made about ageing: the self remains even if the qualities or attributes of personhood and moral agency are subsequently compromised or depleted. But the symmetry is by no means perfect. While age may compromise the attributes of personhood and qualify the extent of moral agency, were age to eliminate some or all of its underpinning attributes, might it not then be possible that personhood (and its moral status) can be lost – through agedness?

In what some have called the new 'neuro-cultures' (Williams et al, 2012), changes in corporeal being have been seen as sources of change in consciousness and mental capacities – hence in the capacity to perform as a self or person. If corporeal changes occur in the ageing brain, including those structures of neuronal functioning that support identity and the self, do these changes imply a diminution of the infrastructure and thereby of the self itself? Or should they be seen rather as part of the ever-changing *external* conditions that the self as a person can and does reinterpret and adjust to – because of its basic 'under-determination' by both its social cultural and biophysical constituents (Sugarman, 2005, p 806)? In other words, should we qualify the symmetry between development and decline, insisting that the processes of acquiring the qualities of personhood are not at all the same as the processes that compromise or degrade personhood and agency? In short, can it not be argued that having become persons we remain persons, and having acquired a moral identity we retain that moral status unless something happens outside the course of normal life (that includes normal ageing).

This leads to an alternative formulation – drawing on the distinction between normal and abnormal change. Does abnormal development or abnormal decline disrupt the continuities of agency and personhood? Is dementia an example of such a disruption? While moral identity may well require evidence of moral agency, perhaps we should distinguish between the two. In making the distinction between agency and identity on the one hand, and identity and status on the other, we can treat the former as evidence of the emergent and evolving human capability to function as a moral agent, while confining the expression 'the moral status of persons' to that of an inherently contingent cultural and social trope. This possibility is explored in the next chapter, when we turn to consider the place of persons and personhood in the social sciences.

Conclusions

As outlined at the beginning of this chapter, our intention in interrogating the notion of personhood is to point out how much more complex it is than seems to be the case at first sight. Kitwood's assumptions about personhood – and those who have pursued person-related models of care – confound metaphysics with moral philosophy, implying that the only conditions threatening adult personhood are those that arise when the circumstances of dementia are transformed by a 'malignant social psychology' (Kitwood, 1997a). By taking the position that personhood is an attribute of relationships, not of capabilities, Kitwood sidesteps any consideration of what we have termed the 'components' of personhood – the necessary and sufficient conditions that render personhood possible. By also treating personhood as a moral status, demanding of certain rights, Kitwood confuses the constitution of personhood with the possibilities for its existence – namely, that it exists in and only in an 'I-thou' relationship. By refusing to consider personhood as an equivalent term for, or constituted by, individual selfhood, agency or identity, Kitwood ends up treating personhood as an abstract, non-agentic moral identity, something that is necessarily 'a valid object of our moral concern' (Ohlin, 2005), and as such, an entity demanding of those rights that follow from it being of moral concern.

While we have no dispute with recognising that people with dementia are and should be objects of moral concern, as, indeed, should any and all people, whatever their disabilities, we also recognise that many people with dementia will lose some – if not most – of the capabilities that have been deemed to constitute metaphysical personhood, such as reflexivity, self-consciousness, second-order volition ('agency-plus', in Taylor's terms) and narrative unity. Such weaknesses may well increase with time. The problem with adopting a personhood-centred approach to helping people with dementia is that it fails to recognise the distinction between these two aspects of personhood, namely, the standing of persons and the capabilities of personhood. By failing to recognise the distinction, this approach risks placing the burden of responsibility on other persons, other selves, to sustain the personhood of individuals with dementia (in the sense of preserving people with dementia's capacities for personhood), as well as sustaining due moral concern for them. Any failure to achieve the former is treated as if it were the inevitable consequence of a failure to realise the latter – what Kitwood termed the product of malign social psychology.

Such problems extend beyond the institutional care of people with dementia. The law, medicine and organisation of health and social care are all deeply engaged in negotiating the significance of moral personhood as well as what constitutes free agency, choice and capacity. That the two ideas of self-as-agent and person-as-status may not be (indeed, should not be) combined, we would argue, should be self-evident. Furthermore, we would argue that neither concept is sufficiently stable to justify their application as criteria that can be applied consistently and fairly to serve the interests of infirm older people with or without dementia, as the interminable debates about the status of moral personhood illustrate (Block, 1995; Rosenthal and Weisberg, 2008; Griffin, 2013). Instead of using the idea of personhood as a fulcrum through which to improve the position of people with dementia (or of other older infirm people in need of care) it might be more helpful to avoid the term (beyond its everyday use, as persons, people, etc). A better stance, we suggest, is to see the solution in terms of negotiating and containing the malign social imaginary of the fourth age, reflexively orienting the moral imperative of care toward such ends. This does not mean neglecting the study of agency, capability, memory, narrative identity or sense of self in people with dementia, and nor does it imply abandoning different ways of supporting such people's existing capacities and minimising any harmful consequences arising from their incapacities.

Whether one chooses to view these problems from a biomedical/chronic illness perspective or from the perspective of 'difference' may not matter so much. What is important is acknowledging that most carers, paid as well as unpaid, are responding to a common, moral imperative of care. They are moral agents. At the same time, the exercise of that moral agency and the social relations of care that embody it may deepen as well as lighten the darkness of the fourth age. To avoid practices deepening its particular imaginary, we suggest, requires no assertions about the 'personhood' of people with dementia, but simply the recognition of a common humanity and the taking of due care by carers as moral agents. In a sense, then, Kitwood was right, because this does mean thinking of persons within social relations, but we would argue that is because care necessarily takes the form of social relations.

THREE

Agency, identity and personhood in the social sciences

In the previous chapter we outlined the various ways that terms like 'agency', 'identity' and 'personhood' have been understood within philosophy, and how such understandings have been applied particularly in response to the problems of mental infirmity in later life. We argued that the de-construction of the term 'person' into the separable issues of agency and identity may provide a more useful framework through which to interpret these problems than by approaches based on the more generic term 'personhood'. Irrespective of their 'powers' to express agency and identity, the common humanity of people with infirmities can serve as the underlying basis for an imperative of care. Late life infirmity and mental decline can be represented as issues of diminished agency as well as disrupted 'identity' without implying any necessary downgrading of the individual's 'personhood' – if the latter is understood as a proxy or placeholder for moral status (that is, that one is deserving of care and concern). While philosophy can help us think more carefully about the problems of mental infirmity in later life, philosophical analyses do not necessarily carry much weight in shaping the everyday practices of care. Neither do they necessarily direct policy-makers and professionals towards better ways of organising systems and structures to support care, carers or the cared for.

In this chapter we turn from philosophical interrogations of agency, identity and personhood to the consideration of these terms from the perspective of the social sciences. Can sociological and/or anthropological approaches to the person prove more useful in better realising the moral imperative of care that we have argued connects social practices to the fourth age imaginary? More distinctly than is the case with metaphysics or moral philosophy, the social sciences are products of their times. It is difficult to ignore the historical development of thinking and writing about 'self', 'identity' and 'agency' in sociology and social anthropology, not least because these disciplines have themselves drawn attention to the geographical and temporal variability shown by such 'discourses' of agency, identity and self-hood (Carrithers, 1985). Before considering the relevance of contemporary social theory to the problem of 'the person' and the moral imperative of care, we begin by exploring how the early pioneers of the social sciences addressed these issues, and in particular, the difficult relationships between 'self' and 'society' and between 'structure' and 'agency'. Although for some contemporary anthropologists and sociologists social structures remain their dominant concern, with the 'self' or 'person' little more than a nodal point within social space and time, for others, agency and identity have become more central considerations in understanding how people make sense of, influence and are in turn influenced by social structures.

As Smith has noted 'there is no social science analysis that does not at least implicitly assume some model of the human to help underwrite its explanation. Therefore the better we understand the human, the better we should explain the social' (Smith, 2010, p 2). But while '... understandings of the human person are foundational to social science theory and research ... sociologists rarely engage in ontological debates about personhood' (Mooney, 2014, p 21). While social scientists were keen to eschew any such metaphysics of the self, from the very beginnings of sociology there were attempts to formulate what might be called 'a sociology of the self' (Burkitt, 1991; Jenkins, 1997; Elliott, 2001; Hodgkiss, 2001). Such attempts, we believe, provide an alternative approach to the problem of personhood and to the moral imperative of care. It is to those beginnings that we now turn.

Durkheimian views of personhood and the self

Although it is customary to see the beginnings of sociological accounts of the self in the work of George Mead and the symbolic interactionist school of the 1930s (see, for example, Elliott, 2001, p 30), concern with the nature and status of the self or person can be traced back to the French sociologist Émile Durkheim's writings of the late 19th century. While such seminal figures as Marx was clearly more concerned with questions of social structure and Weber with processes of individual meaning rather than with the individual per se, Durkheim's thinking about selves and persons developed throughout his professional career. Callegaro has distinguished between the earlier and the later conceptualisation of the person in Durkheim's writing (Callegaro, 2012). In what he called Durkheim's 'weak version' of the individual, human beings are, first of all, human beings filled with personal thoughts and goals; however, until they interact with others they are deprived of all that makes the human a 'social being'. Social being is achieved and true personhood realised only when the individual interacts with others, sharing and pursuing 'collective' ends

(Callegaro, 2012, p 460). This duality of human nature, *homo duplex*, as Durkheim would later call it, was later reformulated in a stronger, more fully social version, in Durkheim's essay on 'The dualism of human nature' (1914/2005). In this essay, Durkheim re-formulates these two aspects of the individual (or the 'two groups of states of consciousness', as he called it), distinguishing the self that is built on the foundation of its body from the self or person who can think, use concepts and reflect on matters beyond his or her corporeal needs, in short, one that is built by society (Durkheim, 2005, p 37). While the latter contains all the necessary conditions of (moral) personhood, the former (the individual reduced to the empirical sensibility of his or her body) lacks the elements of personhood that exist beyond the bare capacity to function as what Dennett called 'an intentional system' (Dennett, 1976).

For Durkheim, the person as a social being also enabled individuals to think 'sociologically', to 'imagine' society by drawing on the collective insight and learning of past and present persons. In Durkheim's mind, this historicity in the development of people as social beings provided the key to thinking sociologically, and nowhere was this process better exemplified than in the work of his nephew and follower, Marcel Mauss. In his account of the evolution of the category of the person, Mauss makes the distinction between what he calls the 'conscious personality' and the 'category of self' (Mauss, 1938/1985, p 3). While a human being's awareness of his [sic] body and 'at the same time his individuality, both spiritual and physical' was seen by Mauss as a universal feature of the species, the category of the self, he claimed, was historically quite recent (Mauss, 1938/1985, p 3). Mauss traces the idea of a self or person from its origins as a role in Greek drama, through the use of the mask, to the use of the status of 'person' as a term in Roman law, and later on to the medieval notion of the person as a unitary, rational being, 'body and soul, consciousness and act' (Mauss, 1938/1985, p 20). It reached its 'latest' (maybe final) transformation into the person as 'self' – the condition of consciousness and 'a being possessing metaphysical and moral value' (Mauss, 1938/1985, p 22).

Like Durkheim, Mauss distinguished between a primary unchanging consciousness or self-awareness and a conceptual awareness of the self. While the former is fundamentally experiential, the latter is necessarily reflexive, the product of collective thinking that has developed over centuries to form the notion of a person as 'self'. Mauss' work maintained that there was a duality between an externalisable 'inner self' that could be explored and understood as 'an other', and a purely internal experiencing consciousness that once animated the role of a person but which now co-exists with its reflexive self. This duality of sense and reflection, subject and object forms a central theme in the 'next' stage in sociological thinking about the self, one framed by a combination of sociology and social psychology in the shape of social interactionism.

From social to symbolic interactionism

If Durkheim located individual selves as inextricably social beings, he did so in order to explain how society worked in and through persons. The person as a social being was a necessary requirement for sociology to become possible as a science, a necessary staging point, and not an end in itself. The first sociologist to treat self-hood as a central focus for social theory was the American, Charles Cooley, in his book, *Human nature and the social order* (Cooley, 1922; Dewey, 1948). Cooley argued that there were two ways of thinking about the self, one as a metaphysical construct 'more or less remote from the "I" of daily speech and thought', and the other 'what psychologists call the empirical self', which, for Cooley, was 'rooted in the history of the human race' and 'defined and developed by experience' (Cooley, 1922, pp 170-1). While he explicitly eschewed any desire to explore the more philosophical aspects of selves and persons, he was eager to explore 'human life' in both its collective and 'distributive' (that is, individualised) aspects.

This empirical or social self was potentially present from birth but formed as a 'consciousness of the peculiar or differentiated aspect of one's life' within existing social relationships (Cooley, 1922, p 179). This consciousness was made up of numerous 'self-ideas' associated with 'self-feeling' that formed 'the intellectual content of the self'. One such self-idea that he considered important was 'the reflected or looking glass self', illustrating the point that who or what we are evolves through the internalised gaze of 'the other', as we learn to see ourselves as others see us (Cooley, 1922, p 184). Although Cooley's ideas about the 'looking glass self' were further developed, by George Mead especially, it is worth noting that this particular facet of the self was for Cooley one idea of self among a variety of other ideas held by individuals, and that the self's view of itself extended beyond the simple reflection of others' views.

Mead himself wrote little for publication. His ideas were collected from lecture notes gathered posthumously by his students and published in a book edited by Charles Morris, entitled *Mind, self and society* (Mead, 1935/1962). Despite the provenance of this book, Mead is now credited with playing a pivotal role in determining how the social sciences approached the question of 'self' and 'self-hood' (Elliott, 2001, p 30). He is seen as the founder of the school of thought that has been grouped together under the term 'symbolic interactionism', whose basic tenet – employed subsequently by Herbert Blumer and others – was that the self or person could be 'split' into two, but not the two selves that Durkheim had in mind (of an animal self and a social being), but two equally social selves – the social agent (or 'I') and the social referent ('me') (Mead, 1935/1962, p 182).

Our 'self', Mead argued, is our consciousness that is itself fashioned from our relationships within the lives of others. What distinguished self-hood for Mead was the reflective capacity that the self develops in the process of becoming conscious. Consciousness involves the acquisition of a sense of self that is both subject (I) and object (me). Through what Mead called 'the turning-back of the experience of the individual upon himself', the individual is enabled to 'take the attitude of the other toward himself', and thereby understand him or her-self as a socially constituted self (Mead, 1935/1962, p 134). This internalisation of the external representations of the individual constitutes the reflexive basis of mind, making minds (and selves) 'essentially social products' (Mead, 1935/1962, p 1). Mead adopts and develops Cooley's idea of the self as a reflexive, 'looking glass self'. Influenced by the Russian psychologist Lev Vygotsky's theory of mental development, Mead considered such reflexivity possible because of language and its role in facilitating symbolic representation. For Mead, it is language, the pro-social tool of human communication, that enables 'the taking over of this external social situation into the conduct of the individual himself [sic]' (Mead, 1935/1962, p 187).

Mead equated the 'I' with social agency, the ability both to act and to react to circumstances, while taking account of the impact of these actions on the self, or socially structured 'me'. It was the self as the socially structured 'me', however, that 'sets the limits ... [and] gives the determination that enables the "I" to use the "me" as the means of carrying out what [ever] is the undertaking' (Mead, 1935/1962, p 210). Without this socially structured self, the agentic self would be unable to act. Individuals as persons are both structured and structuring selves, whose agency is constrained by the internalisation of past and present social interactions. Despite these limiting conditions, the self as an 'I' was nevertheless still capable of achieving change (that is, of acting differently) by making use of and consequently changing this socially structured self. The social interactionist framing of selfhood was further developed by Erving Goffman. In his book, *The presentation of self in everyday life*, Goffman treated the self even more explicitly as social and structured (Goffman, 1959/1971). Emphasising the widespread recognition that people 'play a part' in social life, Goffman insisted that this is more than a common observation, and that 'the very structure of the self can be seen in terms of how we arrange for such performances' (Goffman, 1959/1971, p 244). While he assumed all individuals possess the common habit of enacting their social selves, time and place invariably determine the context and constraints when playing out these roles, such circumstances acting as what Goffman later called the 'framing device' for how the self would be presented in any particular face-to-face encounter.

At this point, the agent engaged in the social presentation of self was generally unexamined, presented merely as 'the individual'. Later in his book, *Stigma*, Goffman introduced the term 'personal identity' to represent the unique nature of a person that exists as a separate yet potentially knowable aspect of a person, one who is distinct from the roles or social identities that he or she possesses (Goffman, 1990). But even this seemingly unique aspect of the person, according to Goffman, remained thoroughly social. First, it represents an 'identity peg' that distinguishes one person from another, whether through their physical features or their behavioural style, whose unique identity is nevertheless capable of being codified or documented. Second, it represents a distinct biography or complex of information about an individual that constitutes a 'unique record' of the person. Finally, Goffman adds that there is a third aspect that 'distinguishes an individual from all others, the core of his being, a general and central aspect of him [sic] making him [sic] different through and through, not merely identifiably different from those who are most like him [sic]' (Goffman, 1990, p 74). This core, however, would remain unexplored by Goffman.

Goffman introduced 'ego identity' as yet another facet of identity. Ego identity, he suggested, represents the 'subjective sense of the person's own continuity and character that an individual comes to obtain as a result of his [sic] various social experiences' (Goffman, 1990, p 129). This sense of self is a 'reflexive' matter, and represents more or less what Mead, and Cooley before him, had called the 'looking glass self' – that internalised, integrated view of oneself as a self or 'ego' that is collated through social experiences of how one has been treated or regarded by others as well as one's own (socially mediated) experience of one's actions and reactions – the ego as a reflexive 'me'. Rather than representing this 'me' as equivalent to selfhood, however, Goffman saw it as but one of a trinity of selves or identities that emerge from growing up and living in society.

Without the notion of a reflexive agentic self, however, it is difficult to make sense of the human agent who is engaged in the various 'face-to-face' interactions that Goffman analyses. Who is 'presenting' his or her social identity to the other? Who is it who is seeking to 'pass' by recalibrating his or her biography or masking some unique identifier of a less than valued identity? Who is it who is selecting, reframing or repeating the various forms of talk – who, if not the self-reflexive agent? While Durkheim, as well as the symbolic interactionists, progressively marginalised the notion of the person as a conscious self and indeed as a self-constituted agent, the related discipline of anthropology went even further, treating the existence of a conscious self as nothing more than a mere historical 'construction' of relatively little value in explaining culture and society (Whittaker, 1992, p 192). The demise and later re-emergence of the self in anthropology provides an interesting and complementary account that we turn to next.

Anthropology: de-centring and re-centring the self

If the symbolic interactionists viewed the self as a combination of 'actor' and 'role', the early anthropologists of the 20th century treated the idea of the self as 'unimportant' to their readings of culture and society. According to Elvi Whittaker, social anthropologists like Radcliffe-Brown insisted that the concept of an individual or person 'was merely a position on the scaffolding of the social structure, devoid of any explanatory power' (Whittaker, 1992, p 192). The idea of the self crept back into anthropology under the influence of Mauss, with his idea of the self being an example of collective thought. Different cultures developed different ways of thinking about or rendering salient the self, and it was as such a purely 'cultural' concept that anthropology first legitimated its interest in the self. From this perspective, it was not so much that individuals were agents or had identities, but that cultures differed in the way they made use of (or failed to make use of) the term 'self' or 'person'.

Anthropological notions of the self were 'relativised' from the beginning, as alternative 'ethno-psychologies'. The study of different selves in different cultures did not take off as a field of interest until the late 1970s/early 1980s, when Mauss' distinction between individual beings as 'bodies' and persons as 'social beings' began to be employed as a way of understanding cultural differences in discourses about selves or persons (see, for example, Fortes, 1973; Middleton, 1973). At the same time that these anthropological discourses about self and personhood developed, they did not attempt to link them to concepts of 'identity' in spite of the fact that the former 'are modelled precisely on the anthropological understanding of identity' (Sökefeld, 1999, p 419). Sökefeld argues that through this curious dissociation of terms, anthropologists were able to 'speak not about the self as an actual reflexive center of the person but only about cultural concepts of such a center', which was a convenient distinction, because, he claimed, 'it relieves anthropologists from giving importance to "actual selves"' (Sökefeld, 1999, p 427). He argued that anthropological conceptualisations of the relation between individual and society needed to 'move away from both social determinism and methodological individualism toward a more dialectical understanding in which individual and society are related by mutual constitution' (Sökefeld, 1999, p 428). Giddens' mid-period sociological work on structuration was proposed as one possible direction for anthropology to follow. Before following up this particular suggestion, however, another point that Sökefeld made is worth noting, namely, that of the relationship between concepts of personhood and structures of power. He suggested that granting or withholding the attributes or even the status of personhood often lies in the hands of those in positions of power, while those with little power may struggle with limited effect to assert claims to any agency or express their identity as persons (Sökefeld, 1999, p 429). While he uses as an example the extreme position of concentration camp inmates, clearly the analogy can be extended to other institutional settings, including those receiving care in nursing homes.

Contemporary sociology and the reflexive turn

When Giddens formulated his 'structuration' approach to sociology in the 1980s, he made 'reflexivity' a central term in his model. Reflexivity, he wrote, is that aspect of human agents:

> ... that is most deeply involved in the recursive ordering of social practices. Continuity of practices presumes reflexivity, while reflexivity is made possible only because of the continuity of practices that makes them distinctively "the same" across space and time. "Reflexivity" hence should be understood not merely as "self-consciousness" but as the monitored character of the ongoing flow of social life. (Giddens, 1984, p 3)

This 'turn' to reflexivity in the social sciences was a further development beyond the representation of self and identity that was espoused by

Goffman and the earlier symbolic interactionists, and which, as Sökefeld has suggested, serves as an alternative to the structural determinism of self-hood espoused by traditional anthropologists.

Reflexivity emerged as a major theme in various disciplines as part of what has been termed the general 'post-modernisation' of the academy (Lawson, 1985). It reflected the growing sense that all forms of knowledge were situated within particular contexts, and thus undermined claims to universal applicability (Lyotard, 1984). Social-psychological and sociological understandings of the reflexivity of the self in the works of Cooley, Mead and Goffman may pre-date these 'post-modern' concerns, but what these contemporary theorists did was to bring the topic of reflexivity to centre stage by articulating it as an explicit element in the relationship between 'self' and 'society'.

In his book, *The constitution of society*, Giddens had distinguished three aspects of agency or 'self-as-an-I'. He proposed a self that functions as 'a basic security system', another self defined by its 'practical consciousness' and a third that is constituted by its 'discursive consciousness' (Giddens, 1984, p 41). In this formulation, he seems to be drawing on the Freudian structures of id, ego and super-ego more than he does on Goffman's social, personal and ego identities. But having established this particular triumvirate he fails to sustain or elaborate on it, adopting, instead, a neo-Meadian position, distinguishing between the individual as 'actor', 'I' and the 'self' (me). He writes:

> The "I" is an essential feature of the reflexive monitoring of action but should be identified neither with the agent nor with the self. By the "agent" or "actor" I mean the overall human subject located within the corporeal time-space of the living organism. The "I" has no image, as the self does. The self however is not some kind of mini-agency within the agent. It is the sum of those forms of recall whereby the agent reflexively characterizes "what" is at the origin of his or her action. The self is the agent as characterized by the agent. (Giddens, 1984, p 51)

At this point, Giddens, it could be argued, had not really gone beyond the position adopted by Mead and the symbolic interactionist tradition. In his later work, he began to explore a different kind of selfhood and reflexivity, operating within the 'discursive' aspects of the self. In doing so he opened up a new avenue to thinking sociologically about self and self-identity, utilising the process of 'reflexive monitoring' that constituted the central agency of actors and that was identified as a major feature of modernity (Giddens, 1990, 1991).

Giddens had earlier outlined three levels of agency: first, self-monitoring and the discursive accounting for actions; second, the unarticulated routinised practices by which individuals orientate themselves towards and engage in social action; and third (and for Giddens the least significant), 'unconscious' motivations and interpretations that reside outside the sphere of discourse and practice that he considered were concerned primarily with 'self-preservation' (Giddens, 1984, p 49). Later, in *Modernity and self-identity*, he claimed that to 'be a 'person' is not just about being a reflexive actor, but having the capacity to use 'I' in shifting contexts – that is, to develop and deploy a 'self-identity'. This is 'the most elemental feature of reflexive conceptions of personhood' (Giddens, 1991, p 53). At this point, Giddens introduces the discursive self as the core of personal identity. Like Goffman's personal self it relies heavily on a continuing narrativity – an autobiographical accounting of self. Rejecting the idea of a 'looking glass self' or a behaviourally styled self, he ends up favouring a self-storying self: 'A person's identity is not to be found in behaviour, nor – important as this is – in the reactions of others, but in the capacity to keep a particular narrative going' (Giddens, 1991, p 54). Such a discursive self-identity requires continuing work, the updating and adapting of autobiography both to maintain coherence with the external world and to ensure continuity between past and present. It also requires what he calls a reflexive biography that he links to the more general phenomenon of developing a trajectory of the self.

Giddens' concept of 'a trajectory of the self' is closely linked to other terms such as the 'life project', 'lifestyles' and 'life plans'. These are all, he suggests, foregrounded in the 'existential terrain of late modern life' where choice and autonomy are valued above all else. In his view, 'late modernity' has created institutions that particularly privilege 'reflexivity', the idea of life as a project, and which encourage every 'I' to elaborate, modify and if need be reinvent the 'me' that is at the heart of the agentic, discursive accounting of one's self-identity. This idea that social institutions foster – or fail to support – individual reflexivity suggests a degree of 'un-freedom' of action, in a philosophical sense, that resonates with the general emphasis within the social sciences on the over-determination of individuals' actions. It has played a particularly important part in the debate over 'reflexive' modernisation and the extent to which individualisation is itself a structural requirement of 'late' modern societies (Beck et al, 1994). Giddens can be seen to reflect a point that Kitwood had made earlier in his critique of dementia, namely, that because modernity has privileged the autonomous production of self, ignoring the relational construction of selves, dementia has come to be seen as particularly demeaning because it represents a loss of this modern Western model of personhood (Kitwood and Bredin, 1992, p 275).

Agency, structure and reflexivity – the work of Margaret Archer

Margaret Archer has provided a more nuanced position regarding agency and reflexivity than that associated with Beck, Giddens and Lash. In a series of works, she has attempted to restore a more central role in the social sciences to the 'I' of agency, at the same time as framing agency within a wider context than the purely social (Archer, 1988, 1995, 2000). Human properties and human powers, she argues, are:

> ... relational: stemming from the way our species is constituted, the way the world is and the necessity of their mutual interaction. The relations between the two, being universal, supply the anchor which moors our elaborated forms as Selves, Persons, Agents and Actors. (Archer, 2000, p 17)

Archer is at pains to replace ideas of agency based on a discursively construed 'self' with the idea of a self that is embodied first and foremost in corporeal action that is only later elaborated within the networks of social discourse. She writes, 'our practical work in the world does not and cannot await social instruction but depends upon a learning process through which the continuous sense of self emerges' (Archer, 2000, p 122). Arguing that 'doings' and not 'meanings' are central to human beings, and that human identity is reducible to neither 'biological bundles of molecules' nor 'society's conversational meanings', Archer seeks to distinguish between 'strict human identity, which makes each of us a unique being' and 'strict personal identity, which makes each of us a unique particular person' (Archer, 2000, p 190). The latter – personal identity – emerges from the self, our embodied human identity, with its 'continuous sense of self'. This emergent property, she argues, depends critically and crucially on 'the activity of the reflective human being' (2000, p 190).

In short, Archer reverses the position of self and agency, crediting the former with being an emergent property of the embodied individual acting and reacting to external reality, while the latter derives from the social context that enables the human agent to function in effect as a person. For Archer, as for Giddens, functioning as a person involves a discursive self or inner conversation that is intimately engaged with and involves participation in social discourse and social practice. Functioning as a person creates the necessary conditions for persons to then become social actors – to enact a social identity. What Archer adds to this narrative is not only the prioritisation of a 'pre-social' self, but also the importance of 'emotion' in animating personal identity. Drawing on another trilogy of terms, Archer distinguishes between three types of interactions between self and 'non-self', which she calls interactions within the natural order, within the performative order and within the social order. Each class of interaction elicits a distinct set of emotions. Thus fear, anger, sadness, joy, disgust and hope are seen as emotions emerging necessarily but not exclusively 'within' the natural order. Their 'location' within the natural order, Archer claims, is 'because such commentaries need make no reference to either material culture or language. The relationship between properties of the environment and of our embodiment are sufficient for their emergence' (Archer, 2000, p 205). The human and social significance of these emotional 'commentaries' lies in their impact on the person as agent, causing the individual to change, continue or cease any particular interactive sequence. Importantly for Archer, their 'location' lies in the natural order 'where the standards for commentary are inscribed physiologically in our organic make up and its capacity to feel pain and pleasure' (Archer, 2000, p 209).

While Archer is less detailed in her analysis of those emotions generated from interactions in the worlds of praxis and sociality, she claims more generally that while these worlds can and do generate the same emotions as those elicited within the natural world, some emotions such as the sense of achievement, failure, shame and humiliation arise necessarily and distinctively from interactions in the worlds of praxis and sociality, respectively. But it is not the fact of these first-order emotions that constitutes the inner dialogue, but their further elaboration that takes place within the inner conversation of the self and that leads to a more articulated elaborate set of 'second-order' emotions. These self-honed second-order emotions express a re-articulation of the first-order emotions through an inner dialogue that 'aligns our predominant concerns with our pre-eminent emotions ... [such that] in this process both elements will undergo modification' (Archer, 2000, p 230). This dialogic process and the resultant second-order emotional commentaries, Archer argues, constitute the richness of the person's inner life. They are necessarily presaged on the emergence of a personal identity, which, in turn, can 'only emerge at maturity once the reflective self had surveyed the full three orders of reality ... and then determined where their ultimate concerns lay' (Archer, 2000, p 257). Social identity represents a parallel but more restricted element of personal identity that is 'only assumed in society' unlike personal identity that 'regulates the subject's relations with reality as a whole' (Archer, 2000, p 257). Archer concludes that if the self stands as the alpha of social life itself, 'the person represents its omega' (Archer, 2000, p 257).

The journey that Archer has taken over these last three decades (1984-2014) reflects more general changes in ways of thinking about the self and personal identity in the social sciences. Of course Archer has had many critics (Caetano, 2015). These include the committed structuralists and their revisionist colleagues who will never concede the privileging of social structures in determining individual and group social interactions, as well as those post-structuralists who refuse to endorse any authorial, let alone agentic, 'unity' to the singularity that she attributes to the self. But if one simply acknowledges that persons or personal selves are more than the pseudo-singularity of 'reflected' selves, personhood must be worth considering as a status that society both recognises and realises. It is not as Mauss and Mead (and in some ways Goffman and Giddens) imply, simply a cultural imaginary concocted to maintain things as they are. This self-realised status of personhood, it can be argued, is evident in the individual's interactions with the natural, the practical and the social world, and equally in the directing influence of the individual's inner dialogue. For Archer, personhood is much more than a discursive self; it is an acting and interacting and, at times, also an agentic self, increasingly directed toward social and moral reflexivity.

Personhood as property and status

If one aspect of the sociological tradition has constructed personhood as performed or narrated personal identity, another has pursued it as a form of status or property, with the implication that individuals can own, lose or be robbed of that property or status by becoming or being designated 'non-persons'. Two writers, Bryan Turner (1986) and Beverley Skeggs (2011), illustrate this position, albeit from somewhat different angles. In his paper on 'Personhood and citizenship', Turner argued that many of the debates and dichotomies within sociological theory were beginning to converge 'on a single issue, which were encapsulated in the notion of "embodied personhood"' (Turner, 1986, p 2). A sociological answer to the question 'what are we?' he states, is 'long overdue'. The category of personhood, Turner suggested, 'is in the process of rapid transformation', a transformation that converts persons into citizens as the successive waves of identity politics stripped 'the multiple layers of particularity' from the individual, rendering the personal political and leaving behind personal identity as little more than 'an empty package' (Turner, 1986, p 14). For Turner, the steady expansion of the public into the private sphere – the intrusion into the domain that Husserl termed 'the life world' – in late modernity is rendering personhood as personal identity an increasingly residual term that is incapable of exercising any social effects (although not, of course, denying personal identity as a source of action 'outside' the public sphere).

In contrast, Skeggs treats personhood as a privileged possession. She argues that the processes of social differentiation in late modernity are leading to extended possibilities of personhood for some, while for others cultural and economic marginalisation is leading them to becoming lesser persons (Skeggs, 2011, p 501). Skeggs writes of 'dominant symbolic circuits of personhood legitimation', whereby some individuals or groups form the '"constitutive limits to proper personhood" – the abject, the use-less subject who only consists of lacks and gaps, voids and deficiencies ... negative value that cannot be attached or accrued and may deplete the value of others through social contagion' (Skeggs, 2011, p 503). Skeggs is arguing here that the 'productivist' model of 'classical' modernity, in which (notionally) everyone was treated as an equal based on their power to sell their labour, has been replaced by an 'equality of exchange', where everyone is deemed equally free to 'produce and publicly perform themselves as "a subject of value"' (Skeggs, 2011, p 508). For Skeggs, as for Turner, personhood is not a function of individual personal identity but a property or status – a reflection of a person's social identity – that is conferred by cultural, economic and social relations. But while Turner laments the loss of the particularity of persons by the overshadowing identity of the consumer citizen, Skeggs protests the new currency by which personhood is judged.

Re-framing personhood as property has been extensively explored within legal studies. Writing in 1982, Margaret Radin noted how 'the relationship between property and personhood ... has commonly been ignored and taken for granted in legal thought' (Radin, 1982, p 957). She considered how personal property might in some way be seen as embodying the person – in short, that property could be viewed as an extension of the self. While it must be accepted that exploring the relationship of self to property is not the same as seeing the self – or selfhood – as property, the connection between these two approaches serves to highlight the potential 'permeability' of both the self and personhood.

In his examination of the nature of 'responsibility' and 'the boundaries of the self', Dan-Cohen raised the question of how issues of responsibility challenge notions of the boundaries – in time and place, and within the social world more generally – of what is 'us' and what 'we' take responsibility or feel accountable for (Dan-Cohen, 1992). He delineates three types of what he calls 'constitutive responsibility' that encapsulate the problem of the self's 'boundaries'. These are responsibility for one's body, responsibility for one's property and vicarious responsibility or responsibility for 'one's people' (that is, one's family, employees, comrades etc). Dan-Cohen suggests that each of these issues demonstrate the 'plasticity' of self-hood, the potential of the self to 'attach or 'invest' itself in things and in relationships and, at other times, to disinvest or detach itself from those same things or persons.

If personhood is a contingent attribute of individuals, dependent on time and place, and capable of being fragmented, graded, sorted or unified according to either social circumstances, corporeal integrity or both, is it necessary, then, to consider personhood as both contingent and normative? How relevant, then, to self-hood or personhood are the criteria proposed by which personal identity is said to be realised, such as the continuity conferred by the capacity for consciousness, communication and memory? How far can one stretch the meaning of agency to encompass both the self as subject and self-hood as status? Might not the agency and identity realised in the interactions within the three worlds that Archer has identified (the natural, practical and social) be different in each case, at different times, and in different circumstances? Nothing in the end may be called unequivocally ours or identified as ourselves, neither through our embodiment, our consciousness, or indeed, our possessions and responsibilities.

Agency, identity, personhood – common themes and points of distinction

David Hume had more or less reached this position of doubt when he felt compelled to question his own understanding of self-hood in an appendix to his *A treatise of human nature*. If, as Strawson has suggested, neither 'pure' consciousness nor 'pure' corporeality constitute our identity as 'selves' since neither exist except as abstract ideas or categories of collective thought, perhaps it is necessary to consider that the self is, as Cooley, Durkheim and Mead have implied, only ever realisable within a social context. In which case, it might be necessary to treat the self and its properties of agency and identity as socially contingent and not as the foundation for human rights or moral status. In other words, there is no realisable self, other than that of the social self. There is no agency other than that of social agency, and there is no identity other than social identity.

If we take on board such a perspective, how should this affect the way we think about agency, identity and self-hood, particularly in the context of later lives affected by illness and infirmity? Given such a necessarily contingent self it could be argued that self-hood ceases to be so problematic. Although agedness, disease and disorder might affect the self's realisation, limit its subjectivity or constrain its agency, they do so in particular ways and in particular circumstances. The constraints on agency, limits to subjectivity and self-realisation should not be seen as simply the inherent basis or consequence of these conditions. Rather than treating mental infirmity as the cause of a loss of agency, the erasure of the person, or the death of the self (Gilleard and Higgs, 2015), it then becomes possible to envisage agency, identity and selfhood as simply less extensive and less stable among individual mentally infirm older people than in the case of less mentally infirm people, and who are therefore in need of more active support.

Identity, agency and personhood may be more or less salient concerns within different environments and in different social relationships. Equally, attributions about these entities may be more or less influential in affecting the narratives and practices of care that in turn depend on how care is itself practised and understood. If, as we have argued, the fourth age is a social imaginary possessed of certain attributes such as frailty, abjection and limited agency, then the more agency is framed in certain ways and given a certain standing (or status), the more likely this particular imaginary will be evoked and socially realised in the narratives and practices of care. The more that a fourth age imaginary is evoked, the more likely it is that any contradictory evidence of identity and agentic power will be ignored or rendered invisible. In contrast, the more that compassion, reciprocity, respect and responsibility are expected, in the context of an older person's mental and physical impairments, the harder it may be to ignore the older person's limited personal agency or fragile identity. At the same time, the more limited an individual's agency and the more fragile his or her identity appears, the more difficult it is for others to sustain the assumption of compassion, reciprocity and responsibility (assumptions that demand ever more emotional and personal effort) and agency from those who are still caring. The idea that the self is simply a notional position or role, a node in a network of obligations and expectations, or a character in a play without authors, should make such efforts to care less problematic. But people are not just nodes, and the social imaginary of the fourth age is frightening precisely because they are not.

Conclusions

The place of terms such as 'agency', 'identity' and 'personhood' remains of continuing interest in the social sciences. The reservations that were expressed earlier by Durkheim, Cooley, Mauss and Mead in the use of such terms still find echoes today. However, in the writings of such contemporary sociologists as Archer, Bauman, Giddens, Skeggs and Turner, these terms are treated as representing meaningful ways of understanding the place of the individual within society. They are not, to use one of Beck's terms, simply 'zombie categories' (Beck, 2001), and nor are they merely convenient cultural imaginaries. As the demands of our time seem to require, individual persons are increasingly reflexive, self-fashioning selves whose second-order concerns and desires are themselves subject to further, third-order thinking, such as exemplified in Archer's category of the 'meta-reflexives'. Consequently, questions of agency and identity have become of central concern within the contemporary canon (Outhwaite, 2009). Having seemingly evolved the capacity for second-order thinking as part of our species being (Marx's '*das menschliche Wesen*'), writers like Archer, Beck and Giddens suggest that contemporary reflexive society is demanding that this capacity shifts up a level. They would argue that there are fewer opportunities and greater costs for individuals deploying over-rehearsed roles within familiar casts in widely known scripts. Instead, our highly individualised societies place ever more demands to adopt third-order meta-reflexivity in our relationships with the social world. While the cultural worlds of the third age may offer opportunities for precisely this type of free play, such self-consciously narrated performances represent the very antithesis of the fourth age's imaginary, where agency seems lost in a kind of black hole (Gilleard and Higgs, 2010), beyond the limits of the personal and the reflexive.

Being persons can never be reduced to simply being bodies positioned in social space, and nor can the self be reduced to the internalised discourse arising from other selves. Pets do not become persons however much we talk to them, give them names, or indeed attribute distinct 'personalities' to them. Being a person, a self, assumes something more – whether that something is framed as self-conscious agency, rationality or reflexive narrativity. To this extent there is consensus between current philosophical and sociological thinking. What sociology has always insisted on, however, is that this 'something more' is thoroughly imbricated within the social and so, by implication, as social institutions and social relations change, so, too, does the nature of selves and persons. An exaggeratedly reflexive society makes for exaggeratedly reflexive selves, and vice versa. Perhaps because of this, dementia and other less profound forms of mental infirmity seem particularly threatening to our contemporary social being.

Once upon a 'pre-modern' time, the fear of old age was largely one of physical decline – the loss of beauty, youth and vitality, of muscular firmness and strength, physical agility, sensory acuity and courage. Such fears expanded (and in part were replaced) in classical modernity to include fears over the loss of earning capacity, the loss of labour power as well as social capital and, by extension, the fear of the loss of one's self as both doer and earner. In Beck's 'second modernity', society is more concerned with the loss of mental power, of the capacity to realise agency, to construct and re-construct identity and to maintain life plans and concerns. We believe that this kind of sociological framework may prove more useful in addressing the dilemmas of persons living under the shadows of the fourth age than questions of either metaphysics or morals, even if the latter provide us with a necessary caution when imagining what care can do.

FOUR

Frailty

The emergence of what has been called a 'hyper-cognitive' society (Post, 1995) and its structural individualisation (Beck and Beck-Gernsheim, 2002) has made the body a key site of identity and embodied difference. The 'corporeal capital' that could be said to be associated with owning a fit body has become a critical resource throughout life (Higgs, 2012). In later life, being fit and healthy enables effective participation in the cultures of the third age, and serves as a key point of reference for older people in judging how well they are doing and how effectively they are managing to age at a distance from the fourth age's shadowy imaginings. For those whose bodies fail to meet these demands, an active mind serves as some form of compensation, demonstrating that despite physical weakness, the individual still has their wits about them. More than other forms of frailty, the prospect of becoming demented represents a major fourth age fear more profoundly than any other infirmity, as it seemingly risks undermining any claim to be ageing well. While the risks of falling, of being unable to walk outside safely, of no longer being able to see or hear clearly pose distinct threats to ageing successfully, the greater threat is that of losing one's ability to represent oneself, not just as 'not old', or 'not past it', but as any kind of valid self or person.

Threats and limitations to exercising embodied agency represent major components of the social imaginary of the fourth age. We have argued that the construct of frailty symbolises those risks (Gilleard and Higgs, 2011a; Higgs and Gilleard, 2015). Geriatric medicine represents frailty as the fulcrum of the specialty, whether conceived of as a distinct syndrome or treated as a symptomatic conglomerate, a condition of cumulative vulnerability and compound risk (Rockwood et al, 1994, 1999; Fried and Walstom, 1996; Fried et al, 2001). Although initially treated as a generic term to replace the use of 'infirmity', biomedical researchers have become committed to viewing it as a multivariate concept, one that is nevertheless capable of being understood, assessed and measured in a manner distinct from diagnosed disease or chronological agedness. The aim of this chapter is to explore how the concept of frailty has come to represent the core of unsuccessful ageing. Framed as a biomedical construct (rather than a biomedical fact), the term (in English, at least) also manages to conjure up the idea not just of physical weakness but also of personal and social 'failure'. Frailty represents the intractable failure of the individual to fulfil the requirements of personhood, of being neither a competent social actor nor embodying a valid social identity. It is scarcely surprising, therefore, that it is an identity few older people would choose to attribute to themselves (Becker, 1994: Kaufman, 1994; Puts et al, 2009).

We examine three aspects of frailty that we feel bear most strongly on this role of 'frailty as failure'. The first is the idea of frailty as a weakened general state and the consequent devalued status of the body associated with that state. The second is the implication of compromised agency and the creation of a vulnerable identity, which raises questions of the extent to which one is one's own person, in particular the ability of the individual to adequately represent themselves as a person in their own right. Third, we would argue, are the attributions of dependency and vulnerability that expose the person, thus 'frailed', to the moral imperatives of care, and the idea that 'something must be done' for such persons. By exploring each of these related aspects of frailty we want to represent it not as a biomedical fact, but rather as a construction with long historical roots (those impotent through age, the 'aged and infirm' etc) that has emerged as if new in the discourses that help realise the social imaginary of the fourth age. In the last section of the chapter we return to the topic of agency, selfhood and identity discussed in previous chapters in order to consider how frailty contributes to and indeed questions their continuing relevance in the deeper recesses of old age.

Biomedical models of frailty

Frailty, whatever else it represents, signals a change in status in later life – one of loss, and the all-encompassing attribution of what can be termed 'frailure'. It has replaced many of the traditional terms once used to describe the sick and vulnerable aged, such as impotence, infirmity or senility. Within the system-world of geriatrics and gerontology, frailty describes people as patients who, without necessarily being diagnosed as 'ill', are nevertheless in a poor way, more vulnerable than those ageing differently, more successfully, and who are judged to lack the power or personal resources to cope with disease, disability and decline (Fisher, 2005, p 2229). In a sense 'frailty' is but another manifestation of the modern infra-structure of 'geriatrics', with its self-defining role in establishing, defending and maintaining 'the distinction between normal old age and senile deterioration' (Hirshbein, 2000, p 346).

Despite attempts at objectifying this state, frailty remains a still 'emergent' construct which, 'like the weather ... resists facile measurement and definition' (Bortz, 2010, p 255). Although recent research consensus has expressed the view that 'frailty has a clear conceptual framework', there is no agreed 'operational definition of frailty that can satisfy all experts' (Rodríguez-Mañas et al, 2013, p 66). Different instruments lead to differing numbers of older people being 'frailed'. One review reported that 'the prevalence of frailty ranged between 33% and 88% depending on the frailty tool used' (van Kan et al, 2010, p 275), while another reported 'enormous' variations in the prevalence of frailty among people over 65 living at home, varying from as low as 4% to as high as 59% (Collard et al, 2012). Even in clinical settings, such as acute geriatric admission wards, where the population might be expected to be more homogeneous, studies have reported rates of frailty varying from 36% to 88% (van Iersel and Rikkert, 2006, p 729).

Much of this variation can be attributed to the scales and criteria used in 'diagnosing' frailty. The more scales used, the greater seems to be the variability. Comparing eight 'commonly used scales' applied to over 27,000 non-institutionalised persons aged 50 to 100, surveyed across 11 European countries, Theou and her colleagues found rates from as low as 6% to as high as 44%, depending on the particular scale (Theou et al, 2013). Another study reported that the proportion of residents in assisted living facilities designated 'not frail' by various 'frailty' scales ranged from as few as 3.5% to as many as 32.3% (Hogan et al, 2012, p 4), leading the authors to conclude that the capacity to predict the 'adverse outcomes', said to define the frail state, 'requires further work' (Hogan et al, 2012, p 8).

The vagueness of the term has not prevented researchers from making frailty a scientifically precise biomedical concept; if anything, it has served as a stimulus for yet more research effort. Within this research endeavour, two lines of enquiry have been followed. One seeks to define frailty as a distinct syndrome or phenotype observed in particular old people distinguishing them from other 'non-frail' old people. This syndrome is judged capable of being identified by a set of discrete 'objective' signs (Fried et al, 2001). The other line of inquiry treats frailty rather less particularly, preferring to frame it as a multi-factorial dimension characterised by various physical, psychological and social characteristics, each observed to varying degrees within any older population. The summation of these 'signs of frailure' assigns older individuals to different positions on an overall scale of frailty representing increasing risk of suffering (yet more) adverse outcomes (Rockwood et al, 1999; Mitniski et al, 2002b).

Measures of frailty based on the former, syndrome approach, have proved capable of distinguishing frailty from related indicators such as 'agedness', 'co-morbidity' or 'disability' (Fried et al, 2001, 2004), suggesting that however vague, frailty can be represented as something other than either functional impairment or disabling ill health. It continues, as it were, to have 'purchase' outside the existing framework of disease or disability. The question remains, however, as to what gives it such purchase. In order to pursue this problem researchers have begun to examine the various constitutive elements proposed to underlie the biomedical concept of frailty, to find which ones 'work'.

When examinations of individual frailty criteria are undertaken, it is clear that not all are equally predictive of adverse outcomes. Single or limited indices seem to be as predictive as more cumbersome, multi-dimensional measures of accumulated deficits. Studies have found that measures of motor activity such as 'slow gait speed', 'low physical activity' or 'lower extremity function' are predictive of falls, chronic disability, institutionalisation and death among non-disabled people over 70 years of age, while self-reported measures of muscle weakness, depression, exhaustion and weight loss are much less predictive (Rothman et al, 2008; van Kan et al, 2010; Vermeulen et al, 2011; Woo et al, 2012). One set of criteria, linked with the so-called Fried phenotype, reflecting muscular weakness and limited physical activity, overlaps considerably with another less widely used term, 'sarcopenia', which, while more narrowly defined and more easily measured, nevertheless lacks the range of application that frailty now possesses.

Frailty as the loss of health reserves

Sarcopenia draws attention to one aspect of age's loss of health reserves – the reduction in muscular definition, loss of muscular mass and limits of muscular power. Unlike frailty, sarcopenia leaves the heart and brain alone. Rockwood, Mitniski and colleagues have argued that unlike such a syndrome, 'the number of deficits, rather than their precise nature, might be the most important determinant' of frailty (Mitniski et al, 2002b, p 5). From this multi-systemic, dimensional perspective, they consider that 'relative frailty and fitness can … be estimated as the difference between chronological and biological age' (Mitniski et al, 2002b, p 7). Understood in this more compound form, frailty covers a broad canvas mapping the terrain between successfully 'ageing on time' and more precipitate forms of ageing, ageing unsuccessfully and before time.

Does frailty represent itself, then, as the loss of physical status and health, as a marker of unsuccessful or frailed age? Or is there more to it than that – does it represent a loss of 'personhood' as well as of social power and status? Is a frail person not just a person with significantly poorer health, but also a failed person, someone not quite up to the criteria of being a full or complete citizen? Fried's syndromal approach to frailty stressed the necessary presence of particular physical symptoms – bodily slowness, weakness and inactivity – but excluded what might be called mental or social ones (Fried et al, 2001, 2004). Rockwood, on the other hand, included mental symptoms as integral to its definition (Searle et al, 2008; Pel-Littel et al, 2009). Research exploring the association between mental impairment and Fried's syndromal approach to measuring frailty has found clear connections between these phenomena (Panza et al, 2006; Boyle et al, 2010; Buchman et al, 2007; Garcia-Garcia et al, 2011; Shimada et al, 2013), leading some to argue that 'cognitive impairment is a clinical feature of frailty and … should be included in [its] definition' (Kulmala et al, 2014, p 16). Others have called for a new form of frailty, termed 'cognitive frailty' (Panza et al, 2007; Kelaiditi et al, 2013; Woods et al, 2013), which can be added to the catalogue of forms of frailty, that might also include forms of social frailty or vulnerability (Andrew et al, 2008). With age, the number of people who are labelled physically frail increases, as do the number of people who are mentally (or cognitively) frail. So, too, it appears do indicators of social frailty or vulnerability. Might it not be simpler to argue that the longer one lives, the more likely one is to be labelled mentally, physically and socially 'frail'? This is perhaps unremarkable, reflecting little more than the observation that ageing is a deleterious process, affecting some people more than others, and affecting people more the older they get. Might it not be more parsimonious to dispense with the dichotomy between ageing and disease, and acknowledge that with more age comes more pathology and with more pathology, growing impotence and a concomitant decline in status and power? Rather than thinking of there being two categories of person in later life – the fit and the frail, the successfully and unsuccessfully aged –might it not make more sense to consider later life as a minefield strewn with increasingly disabling dangers and diseases that gets harder to navigate the longer the journey and the older an individual gets.

By thinking of these dangers and diseases as 'disabling' it becomes possible to consider the potential value to be drawn from studying frailty as a form of disablement, in which the process of labelling risks placing further disadvantages in front of the 'frailed' person, by compromising their identity as 'old and frail' or 'at risk', and further hobbling their potential for agency by drawing attention to and increasing the potential adversity of those circumstances from which the frailty narrative derives its 'corporeality'. Even in the presence of frailty and vulnerability – at least as judged by professionals – most older people are reluctant to seek out formal care services in part because of such fears of being 'frailed' by them (Themessl-Huber et al, 2007). Just as wearing a hearing aid risks spoiling one's identity as a competent, able-bodied adult, even more so does the risk of being frailed threaten the identity of older people – as in those circumstances when a call bracelet is attached to the person's wrist, or an alarm is placed round their neck, or their car keys are taken away, or a 'care plan' is written out and kept on the kitchen table for other 'carers' to consult. Frailty becomes a symbol of impairment and insufficiency, a public signifier of risk that implicitly or explicitly reduces the freedom of action and the authority of the older person, who is thus disabled both as citizen and consumer.

Frailty: compromised agency/flawed identity

The losses associated with frailty are compounded by a decline in status. The processes of frailing constrain the freedom of the person – both by external means and by the internalisation of fears that have themselves become pervasive presences in later life. To what extent does frailty result in social disadvantage, and to what extent does social disadvantage make real the adverse outcomes frailty purports to predict? Starting with the first question, it seems that there is quite consistent evidence of a positive relationship between indices of frailty and variously measured indicators of 'social vulnerability' (Andrew et al, 2008). Such associations have led to rather different responses.

Some have used this evidence to argue for an ever more inclusive conceptualisation of frailty that incorporates 'losses in one or more domains of human functioning (physical, psychological, social), which is caused by the influence of a range of variables' (Gobbens et al, 2010, p 356). This expanding catalogue of negative outcomes seems to return frailty to its earlier framing as those 'impotent by age', whose failure to provide for themselves, whether due to physical or mental infirmity, a lifetime of intemperate habits, or the limitations of bare subsistence required some collective provision of care in the form of the workhouse and associated infirmaries. This expansion of the field of frailty that encompasses body, mind and social being reinforces the person's status as 'indigent', 'destitute' and 'dependent', and in effect places them among the abject poor. Others have taken a different position, arguing that it is the mean conditions of the person's life before they grew old that renders them frail in their old age. 'Unsuccessful' ageing is seen as the culmination of 'un-success' throughout life, and frailty the culmination of a lifetime of cumulative disadvantage. Although this line of research can be related to the wider literature on 'health inequalities' in later life (see, for example, Majer et al, 2011), its extension to the field of frailty has been held back by the dominance of frailty as a distinct 'geriatric syndrome'. This has effectively kept it at a distance from both the sociology of health and from social models of disability.

Support for maintaining a distinctly age-related view of frailty can be found in a number of studies. In one Spanish epidemiological study, Garcia-Garcia and colleagues found that while frailty was associated with increasing age and disability, it was unrelated to either past occupation or education (Garcia-Garcia et al, 2011). A similar lack of association with income and education was reported in the US by Hirsch and colleagues, although these latter authors did find differences in rates of frailty by 'race', with older African Americans being significantly more often assessed as frail compared with their white age peers (Hirsch et al, 2006). Other studies indicate that the prevalence of frailty varies systematically with present income and past education, such that poorer people with less education are more likely to be classified as frail as are people who rent (rather than own) their home and people who report a less secure income (Szanton et al, 2010; St John et al, 2013; Woo et al, 2005).

How far social vulnerability is conceptualised as either a component of frailty or a cause or a consequence depends on both the reading of the literature and the orientation of the study. There is evidence to suggest that self-ascription of frailty is integral to older people's social withdrawal and disengagement (Puts et al, 2009; Warmoth et al, 2016), but such findings are based on cross-sectional research that confounds cause and effect. Longitudinal studies seeking to determine who becomes frail (or who gets to be termed frail) may have different antecedents, depending on whether such attributions are accepted and internalised by the older person him or herself, and to date, most research objectifies frailty and in so doing includes within that identity many who would challenge or reject the term. So long as it is framed as a biomedical fact, rather than a construct employed in geriatric and gerontological research, no resolution is likely; such ambiguity only helps foster a deeper and darker imaginary of the fourth age as a process of othering.

Frailty and the moral imperative of care

The idea that frailty comes from within, that it is an endogenous product (or by-product) of ageing, rather than a status derived from external processes, positions it in a rather different and potentially more universal social space. Frailty as the end point of a universal process like ageing makes it seem a point which we can all expect to reach. This viewpoint carries with it a clearer imperative that we should care for those who are frail, since, sharing Rawls' 'veil of ignorance' (Rawls, 1985), we all face the likelihood that we, too, will age, and by ageing, become frail. Unlike the almshouse, poorhouse or workhouse infirmary, the nursing home as the home of frailty seems a less contentious institution, a final destination as democratic as the grave (Ahmad and O'Mahony, 2005; Houttekier et al, 2011; Broad et al, 2013; Reich et al, 2013; Hedinger et al, 2014).

But the internalised state of frailty is not always accepted as a necessary end-product of ageing. Indeed, research suggests that irrespective of their age or health, most older people actively resist frailty as an identity (Warmoth et al, 2015). Reasons for resistance seem to cluster into three general positions. First, that the term implies some kind of moral failing – a submission to the body's weakness that implies a lack of determination or will power (Puts et al, 2009, p 263); second, that it implies a state of depression or demoralisation as if becoming frail is the result of suffering multiple trauma (Puts et al, 2009, p 262); and third, that it represents the embodiment of previous bad habits and mistaken choices, whether as lifestyle failure, inactivity, poor diet, or self-neglect (Puts et al, 2009, p 263). Those who do succumb to self-identifying as frail seem to focus instead on the things they can no longer do – in effect, choosing to see themselves as less able, less active because of processes of ageing decay or deteriorating health (Warmoth et al, 2015). Acknowledging incapacity seems to also acknowledge dependency, needing the help of others, while resisting a frailed identity represents an assertion of autonomy and independence.

Not that the assertion of autonomy means that receiving help from others is automatically resisted or rejected. Other identities, particularly those based on the moral identities of family, enable older people to expect assistance, company or help from their partner, children or siblings, and do not position them necessarily as frail. Negotiating this position between wanting help – needing assistance – and being incapable or incapacitated is clearly not an easy position, but as Grenier and Hanley have noted, some older people can subvert their self-identification as frail while employing the social attributions of frailty to obtain services or other resources without internally accepting oneself as 'abject' or 'frail' (Grenier and Hanley, 2007, p 219).

In short, the link between dependency/frailty and the moral imperative for care leads to four potential outcomes for older people with disabilities: the rejection of frailty as an identity and any need for care; the rejection of frailty but with the expectation of care as help from others; the use of frailty as a means of accessing help not otherwise offered, but without the internalisation of the identity; and the acceptance of frailty, dependency and care. It is difficult to believe that, of all four possible stances, this latter position is not the most harmful to the person adopting it. But is that always the case? A person who believes they can look after themselves perfectly well, may, nevertheless, live in squalor, appear 'abject' in others' eyes and be at constant risk of serious harm, injury or malnutrition. It ought to be possible to accept one's incapacities and still reject being 'othered' by frailty – in short, to need and expect help without that compromising one's agency or sacrificing one's autonomy. Frailty is constructed as a binary; dependency as a matter of degree, and accepting a degree of dependency may be less damaging than accepting the uncompromising identity of frailty.

Gerontology has a history of attempting to reframe the concept of dependency, to make of it a less belittling term (Post, 2006). These attempts have ranged from the acknowledgement of lifelong human inter-dependency, whose forms and expression vary systematically across the life course, to the acknowledgement that growth and decline are intrinsic components of being human life and necessitate social institutions to ensure the reproduction of social life (Munnichs, 1976; Phillipson et al, 1986; Johnson, 1995). The disability rights movement sought to more radically reframe dependency as a creation of social policy, and as a response to the rise of industrialisation (Oliver, 1989). In this they echoed the social dependency theories of earlier social gerontologists (Walker, 1980; Townsend, 1981) who also claimed that representing older people as dependents was a function of pension policy, institutionalisation and community care practices.

These positions inevitably clash. On the one hand are those who argue that 'independent living' is possible for everyone, providing only that society invests in improving access and removing barriers to the full inclusion of people with physical or mental impairments. On the other are those who claim that independent living, in the sense of depending on no one to live and sustain one's life, is impossible, and that inter-dependence characterises all social beings throughout life (Smith, 2001). Dependence is either normal and natural or it is not: there seems little scope for compromise. Just as frailty can seem an identity imposed on some older people in order to organise health and social care services, reinterpreted as vulnerability, frailty can be seen as a universal feature of our whole species, forever at risk of harm, injury and death, forever frail.

Arguably the moral imperative of care serves a dual function, creating the expectation of help while distinguishing the fit from the frail, the needy from the needed. Acknowledging that one has needs is not the same as being labelled 'needy'; acknowledging that one has limitations is not the same as being labelled 'limited'. The narratives and practices of care arise in response to perceptions of lack and need, but they also arise from the desire to help, to remove lack and reduce need. The frustration of those whose needs go unheard is matched by the frustration of those whose care fails either to resolve the lack or meet the desires of those to whom that care is directed. Frailty reflects the latter – a vulnerability that cannot be fully guarded against. It ignores the desires that are not met, until there are no longer any desires, only needs. Internalising frailty as an identity is more than simply acknowledging one's limitations, one's dependency; it implies replacing the desire for living with the necessities for sustaining life.

Conclusions

Frailty, or rather the construct of frailty, is central to the fourth age imaginary. Although the term has come to be used as a biomedical construct whose meaning can be operationalised through ratings and scales, it retains an irredeemable ambiguity, one that no amount of empirical research or clinical investigation can resolve. In this chapter, we have tried to highlight three themes that we think underlie the concept of frailty. First is its use in representing the loss of what could be described as corporeal capital – the physical and mental integrity that serves as the resource enabling us to be what we want to be and to do what we want to do, a loss of potential and of capability. The second refers to the loss of embodied agency and the capacity to represent our bodies as our selves, as distinct social beings capable of expressing distinct social identities, the loss of agency and identity. Third, frailty embodies the idea of dependency and a need for care, and with it the potential loss of autonomy.

Each of these themes overlaps with and yet contains distinct aspects of personhood. Loss of health and capacity involves a shift from the cultures of the third age where ageing can be successful into the social imaginary of the fourth age where assessment of failure abounds, and where there seems to be only one direction of travel. The loss of embodied agency compounds this dependency by ultimately leading to social exclusion and a flattened two-dimensional identity separated from past selves and past social distinctions. Finally, frailty represents the very essence of physical and often cognitive dependency where the person is located mainly through the third person narratives of social and health care professionals as well as by others. The person under these circumstances becomes a shadow of the 'real' personhood enjoyed by others; indeed, it almost seems to exist to demonstrate that difference.

FIVE

Understanding abjection

If frailty has come to signify the vulnerability of older people, abjection reveals the distaste associated with such frailty. In the past, as long as charity was in part a matter of conferring spiritual benefits onto potential donors, the cause and character of the recipients' impoverishment was largely irrelevant. When poverty and dependency represented the collective fate of so many of the common population, the presence of so many poor provided a ready means by which elites could add spiritual value to their existing material resources (Himmelfarb, 1984; Fraser and Gordon, 1994; Jütte, 1994). This pre-modern 'sacral' view of poverty began to change, and from the 15th century onwards poverty's social imaginary was redrawn. Rather than the poor being considered all equally God's children, the communal equivalent of a suffering Christ or *pauperes Christi*, poverty became castigated and thereby categorised into the 'deserving' and the 'undeserving'.

Although it is almost impossible to prove, recent reviews of pre-reformation charity suggest that it may well have been more extensive and more comprehensive than was previously assumed (Rushton, 2001; Dyer, 2012). One consequence of the social disruption of the 'Black Death' in 14th-century Europe was a reduction of poverty's spiritual dimension and a correspondingly greatly increased interrogation of those who were deemed its temporal representatives (Mollat, 1986, pp 251-9). In the process of what has been called the 'desacralisation' of the poor, those deemed 'undeserving' were denied support and were instead criminalised, subjected to persecution and whenever possible, made to suffer (Geremek, 1997). The suffering of the deserving poor was the only kind of poverty that was meant to be relieved, and this was done in a more discriminating manner than before. Poor relief took on a greater variety of institutional forms ranging from the granting of licences to beg to the establishment of almshouses, asylums, hospitals and poorhouses. Meantime, beating and branding, bridewells and imprisonment became common responses to those categorised as the 'shameless poor'.

The shame attached to poverty became accentuated. Even the mendicant religious orders were criticised for being 'worms living in idleness off others' labour' (Mollat, 1986, p 297). As the legislation of the time formalised the distinctions between different groups of poor people, hatred and fear of the vagabond became the antithesis to pity for the orphan and the widow. With the growth of towns and cities, the roaming poor became a greater threat to those with property and power. Such rootless poverty was perceived as alien and dangerous to society rather than an inherent part of it. Even so, within the constraints of a largely agricultural economy, the rise of an abject class would take some time to form, and throughout much of this early modern period, the poor remained a more or less manageable group.

Until the late 18th century, the majority of paupers in Europe (that is, those receiving some form of official relief) were children and old people (Jütte, 1994, pp 40-1). The numbers of adults 'of working age' who received poor relief rose or fell with changes in the agricultural economy. Then came the upheavals of urbanisation and industrialisation. If the de-sacralisation of poverty and the accompanying distinction between the deserving and the undeserving poor had been highlighted earlier by the rise of humanism and the stringencies of the Protestant reformation, the subsequent recalibration of poverty was a product of the industrial revolution and the rise of an urban labour market. The relatively stable rural economies that had been subject to 'natural' variation in harvests and crop failure were now transformed into dynamic, urbanised industrial nation states. There were few alternatives for most people except work and wage labour. As the necessity to sell labour grew in importance, a much narrower and sharper focus on poverty was framed as the inability or unwillingness to exchange labour power for an income.

The lack of paid work defined the pauper and, in itself, became a source of shame. The more flexible, localised and personalised systems of relief practised in the 17th and 18th centuries were replaced by more invariant, institutionalised systems of poor relief such as that typified by the workhouse. Nineteenth-century poverty, like labour itself, was now a matter to be measured, mapped and its causes subject to statistical analysis (Goldman, 1991). A new distinction was introduced between the poor and the destitute. The former earned little and saved little but most of the time managed to survive on their earnings. The latter earned nothing, saved nothing and could only survive by receiving assistance or by resorting to other, criminal means. This line between the pauper and the poor, separated the lower classes, the class of independent labourers, from the abject classes, the 'lumpen' or residuum (Himmelfarb, 1984, p 163). For writers such as Marx, the abject or lumpen were the rabble, the residuum of all classes lacking any collective interest or any capacity for social integration, their political actions more often serving reactionary rather than radical ends (Marx, 2002).

Others, writing from quite different perspectives, were more concerned with this distinction than Marx, for whom the *lumpenproletariat* was a subject of passing interest in the study of the history of class struggle. Writers such as Edwin Chadwick and Nassau Senior, however, were concerned with formalising a clear dividing line between the 'decent' and the 'destitute', and in devising the most appropriate means of supporting the one while disciplining the other (Englander, 2013, pp 10-12). Although the categorisation of the abject proceeded, in the British Isles at least, through the state's formulation of the 'new Poor Law' and subsequent provisions for able-bodied unemployed men, orphaned or abandoned children, deserted or fallen women, sick and disabled people, as well as for the aged and infirm, the greatest concern was for the former – the undisciplined, able-bodied pauper. As the industrialised nations advanced, however, the nature of the state's moral imagination turned increasingly toward considerations of welfare and reform (Himmelfarb, 1991).

The 19th century became an era for all manner of classifications and categorisations applied equally to the social as to the natural world. These statistical efforts produced new information about occupations and illnesses, household structures, ages and education of the whole population which, in turn, led to an intensified search for the causes of society's problems (Dean, 1991; Higgs, 2004). Diseases were classified, occupations categorised, poverty measured, public health assessed and the chronology of the life course recalibrated by a series of laws that effectively institutionalised working life as a fixed period from 14 or 15 to 60 or 65 (Anderson, 1985; Held, 1986). These new methods of statecraft, or 'police science', to use Foucault's term (Curtis, 2002; Foucault, 2007), with their emphasis on economic and social calculation and the numerical ordering of society, facilitated the emergence of various institutional provisions intended to address some particular aspect of disease, disability or disorder. Although welfare in the Victorian period may seem to have been dominated by the workhouse as *the* structure for disciplining the abject classes, both in the British Isles and in other countries across the world, new institutions were appearing, ranging from district and specialist hospitals and infirmaries, to specialist mental asylums, epileptic colonies and industrial schools where pauper children could be taught a trade. Each of these developments was accompanied by the emergence of a new middle class oriented toward public service (Perkin, 1990).

Despite the proliferation of such institutional and professional resources, most countries still relied on general all-purpose institutions for the destitute of all classes, ranging from harmless lunatics to the chronic sick, the aged and the orphaned child. But as the position of the abject classes became more regulated, some of the fear and distaste surrounding the workhouse and its inmates began to be replaced, or at least supplemented by a more sympathetic concern for their plight as part of what Himmelfarb has called 'the moral imagination of the late Victorians' (Himmelfarb, 1991). No longer were the destitute the focus of condemnation or condescension. The very abjection of their incarceration became a matter of public shame. As the statecraft of statistics was brought to play to de-toxify these houses of destitution, the parameters of pauperdom, its causation and consequent possibilities for amelioration became topics of critical political and public debate.

By the beginning of the 20th century, the problem of abjection, identified as that level of abject poverty that persisted across the wealthiest of nations, ceased to be a matter of personal shame and became one of public concern. The abjection of destitution was a matter thought capable of elimination, by new labour laws, by systems of social security, and by more extensive healthcare, with the state acting as the main agent of reform. The 'people of the abyss', as the writer Jack London had called them (1903), were no longer left to the trials of the workhouse and its criterion of 'less eligibility'. The task of reducing and eliminating rates of 'abject poverty' fell to a new generation of moderns, and the concept of an abject class would slowly fade from consciousness (Rowntree, 1901, 1941; Rowntree and Lavers, 1954).

The fate of the abject class

The notion of 'an abject class' re-emerged as a narrative theme in the reception to a short essay written by Georges Bataille in the early 1930s, but which was not published until after his death, in 1972. It was not translated into English until 1999 (Bataille, 1999). By this time, the term 'abject' had already been appropriated by cultural and literary studies following the publication of Julia Kristeva's book, translated as *Powers of horror: An essay on abjection* (1982). Her psycho-analytic use of the term had by far the greater influence on subsequent academic discourse, both in the humanities and in the social sciences, than did the formulation of Bataille. Although Bataille had himself made use of Freudian terminology, the thrust of his essay had been less on the psychic nature of disgust than on the existence of an abject class and its peculiar interdependence with society's dominant ruling classes.

Drawing on both Marx and Freud, Bataille defined the abject class by their inability to escape from abject ('shitty') circumstances, at work and at home. Bataille further argued that this position of abjection held a hidden potential for transgression – a power he believed that could be turned against those who kept the abject firmly in their place in the gutter. In this he moved beyond Marx who held no hope for the *lumpenproletariat* to serve anything other than reactionary ends.

In a sense Bataille was returning to the early modern concept of 'vagabondage' and the able-bodied beggar who threatened to overturn the power and position of their betters. Bataille's work takes up where Marx's ended in *The Eighteenth Brumaire* while raising the potential value of the abject to affect change for, and by, themselves. His position is evident in another earlier essay he wrote exploring the nature of fascism (Bataille, 1979). In this essay, he considered the distinction between what he termed the heterogeneous elements in society and those groups that formed society's homogeneous classes. The latter were seen by Bataille as being homogenised by the ordered relations of production – essentially, the property-owning bourgeoisie and the industrial proletariat. Bataille's heterogeneous elements were made up of two distinct yet related groups – the first defined by 'superior heterogeneity' such as that demonstrated by the fascist leaders and the military, who were everything and yet nothing, who realised their power by uniting and regulating the formless heterogeneous elements making up an army, who transformed the mob into 'a purified geometric order … [of] … aggressive rigidity' (Bataille, 1979, p 78). The second grouping – at the opposite end of society – was made up of 'those who generally provoke repulsion and cannot be assimilated by the whole of mankind' (Bataille, 1979, p 71). These 'fundamentally' heterogeneous elements were the truly destitute who functioned in ways that Bataille likened to the 'untouchable' castes in India, whose 'vile forms' he would later recast as the abject classes. Their 'impurity', Bataille argued, could either be rendered pure by the ritual of their militarisation within the fascist organisation, or be turned upside down by such themes as the pre-modern notion of 'sacred poverty' (Bataille, 1979, p 71).

Bataille's abjection forms both a bridge and a barrier between these invariably fragmented social forms. On the one hand, it contrasts the dangerousness of the able-bodied *lumpenproletariat* with the deservingness of the aged infirm (along with their very different potential for affecting social transformation). On the other, it outlines a common position occupied by all those unable to escape from life's 'shittier' aspects, people removed from and marginal to the ordered relations of production. What differs is their respective danger and risk, their potency and impotency, their scope for agency. Even if 'little old women' can at times play on their status of 'frailty', much like beggars can play on their limblessness or senselessness, the risks of such performances is that they compromise any subsequent return to positions of social agency. Even such performativity as is possible functions primarily within the realm of an unequal exchange – between supplicant and official, patient and doctor, dependent and carer. Unlike people with disabilities, the 'impotent aged' remain an abject class defined by a lack of collective voice and an unfashionably unalterable vulnerability. Left to themselves, their abject status further corrodes their social agency; their lack of physical financial and social power renders them impotent to resist the conditions of their care (Gilleard and Higgs, 2011b). All that is left, it seems, is for the impotent aged to be re-presented, as Bataille suggested, as *pauperes Christi*, which now, in a more secular age, translates as the 'carriers of humanity's inherent vulnerability' (Turner, 2006, 2009).

If Bataille's radical use of the term can be seen as a response to the rising intolerance of the 1930s and the threats posed by fascism and national socialism, the outcome of the Second World War and the subsequent development in both East and West of systems of social protection and social security saw abject poverty receding in significance, whether conceived as a threat to, or an indictment of, society. There was a shift in focus, away from absolute to relative poverty, and with it a decline in the extent to which old age was understood through its impotence and impoverishment. In one of the first, transnational studies of the status of old people in modern society, published in 1968, one of the authors concluded that while 'most old people are fairly securely knitted into the social structure', they are treated as 'a distinct social stratum or category ... a kind of potential or embryonic "class" accommodated uneasily in the present class structure' (Townsend, 1968, pp 425-6).

It is difficult to know exactly what kind of an embryonic class Townsend foresaw emerging. If one tracks the progress of retired people – or pensioners – over the course of the last half-century, their relative poverty, whether measured in terms of income or consumption, has declined, compared with other age groups (Belfield et al, 2014; Jenkins, 2015). Although there are significant social divisions within later life, the evidence for viewing pensioners or retired people, en bloc, as an economically 'excluded class' is fast fading away. Debates about poverty, its measurement and categorisation have been replaced by concerns over social exclusion, a related but nevertheless distinct term that focuses less on income and wealth and more on the deprivation of access to and engagement with all those aspects of life that constitute living well and feeling part of society. What seems to be emerging is a new divide in later life, between the socially engaged and included retiree and the excluded other, whose privatised otherness is a function neither of income nor of wealth but of their lack of agency, capability and identity. This new divide separates people in later life into two classes – the fit and the frail, the agentic and the abject – a divide that overwrites other more conventional social divisions in later life (Gilleard and Higgs, 2016).

The workhouse once served as the institutional representation of the abject classes; they were defined by their impotence and impoverishment, and by their lacking the familial and financial resources to sustain body hearth and home. What has replaced the workhouse, in the 'postmodern' landscape of the 21st century, is the nursing home. While the middle classes were more or less unaffected by the dread of the workhouse in first modernity, the fear of ending up in a nursing home affects equally the retired banker, the retired builder, the retired shop worker and the retired doctor. This is the dubious democratisation of the fourth age's imaginary. While money and family connections once kept such fears at bay, no other source of power or agency can now seemingly combat such fears beyond the dubious distinctions of the body and its precarious status as fit or frail.

Frailty as a marker of a new abject class

In the previous chapter we explored the role of frailty in representing the boundaries of the fourth age imaginary and its multi-dimensional meanings as physical, psychological and social capital, and the extent to which it represented a contested status, one attributed to and resisted by older people themselves as not serving their interests. While physical incapacity may draw such attributions from others, mental capacity can be an important counter-weight – the ability to articulate alternative more positive identities and to contest attributed more negative identities. When mental combines with physical frailty, the person moves from occupying a domain of being capable of at least potential agency to a state of thorough abjection. It is an attributed status of otherness excluding agency because it is determined by the attributions of others, no matter what the person so judged might feel, think or wish, precisely because the judgement of mental frailty or incapacity means others are necessarily better placed to determine the person's objective interests. While this state of abjection arises in and through social relations, as did the abject classification of the impotent aged, the social relations of the abject in second modernity are more thoroughly one-sided and irredeemable. For them there can be no stories of redemption through the introduction of the state pension or the ministrations of the post-war geriatricians. The inability of the 'frailed' person to appear as a clean, capable and competent citizen is a sign of their abjection precisely to the degree to that it is evidenced in and through the eyes of those whose agency and powers of attribution are unquestioned.

For those who witness the abject state of elderly frail or disabled people, it is commonplace that they demand that 'something must be done'. While it may not be clear precisely what must, or can, be done, such cries call on a moral imperative for collective others – family, neighbours, local or national government – to act. What determines the nature of this response are the very signs of abject frailty. These are many and various, depending in part on the 'position' of the individual frail older person. Those that arise during the process of someone's frailty coming to the attention of 'others' will differ from those that arise after the person has already been deemed potentially or actually frail, while others may arise that threaten to further categorise the older person as no longer simply 'infirm' or 'impotent' but 'incompetent' in the sense of lacking capacity to judge their own interests, let alone perform their own self-care. Such signs as these are not controlled by the person but rather are leaked, without their knowledge or consent, and, no doubt, against the person's wishes. The person's impotence to 'unfrail' themselves, to recover or restore his or her state as an agent, then renders the person doubly abject, having become 'irretrievably' frail.

While these signs of abject frailty are typically interpreted as the frail or disabled person being at risk of physical harm and/or personal disaster unless others act on his or her behalf, there usually exists another equally strong but opposing desire not to interfere, not to risk limiting or constraining the person's freedom. No doubt there are distinct cultural and social differences in how such balancing of obligations are to be calibrated, but it seems that there are few circumstances when no such set of conflicting rules apply. Assuming that the obligation to engage is greater than the obligation to leave well alone, we must ask, what consequences flow from the overriding of agency of the infirm person by the agency of the helping other?

In the first place, the activation of the deed – the something that has to be done – effectively constrains the agency of the person to whom help is given, while enhancing the agency of the person helping (or caring). But when the situation is repeated, when it becomes regularised or institutionalised within the practices of care, does that lead to a progressive widening of the 'agentic' gap between helper and helped, carer and cared for? We would suggest that it does not. By repeatedly positioning oneself as 'obliged', there is no sense that the carer or helper gains ever greater agency, nor any sense of 'empowerment', because each something to be done only deepens the need of the deed. The older person's infirmity, impotence or frailty is not lessened by the help given and is not neutralised but enhanced and sharpened by care. While parents or caregivers might generally anticipate helping the child they care for become progressively more independent, frail older people are not children; they are not growing up but growing older, and likely growing more frail. Practices of care enchain further practices of care; the network of care tightens around both the carer and cared for, and agency is corroded.

Of course, it does not always happen like this. When the old man falls while crossing the road, or the old woman falls as she gets out of her car, and a passer-by hurries to help and check that everything is okay, the shadow of the fourth age, the glimpse of abjection, passes quickly. Neither helper nor helped are seriously harmed, although the agency of the helped may be hurt, and that of the helper momentarily enhanced. The potential shame of 'the body drop' can be recovered (McKee et al, 2005). But for some, such incidents become increasingly frequent – frequent falls, frequent 'frailures', leading to frequent calls for something to be done establish a set of obligations around which the networks of care gradually emerge. Within this set of obligations come new narratives and practices of care that define a different set of social relations, just as the beggar at the door becomes an ever regular visitor and subsequently an ever more onerous guest.

Abjection's dirty work

As Bataille was well aware, there is a close connection between abject classes and abject work. Those who spend their working lives picking through refuse dumps for plastic or metal that can be recycled are widely considered to be doing society's dirty work, and are thought to do such jobs precisely because they are among society's most destitute (Gregson et al, 2014). At some point, care for infirm old people began to constitute dirty work – the work carried out in almshouses, hospices and workhouse infirmaries, often by paupers themselves, or 'pauper nurses' who could be as old, if less infirm, as those to whom they tended. This status was not always ascribed to care work. In the genteel almshouses established during the late middle ages and early modernity, the aged residents seem to have been well looked after, as were the aged hospice inmates who were typically cared for by religious orders or other servants of the church, when these and other related institutions were generally small, not exclusively designed to house the most infirm and wretched, and were usually overseen by an order that sacralised the care of the sick and the poor.

Although charitable homes for the aged and infirm existed in both Europe and North America, by the 19th century, most institutional provision for the aged poor provided little more than the warehousing of aged and infirm paupers, with poor care generally delivered by an ill paid workforce. Echoes from this latter tradition affects today's care sector much more than the earlier 'pre-modern' forms of sacral care. Student nurses' attitudes toward working with older adults tend to be negative (Courtney et al, 2000; McLafferty and Morrison, 2004; Gallagher et al, 2006), as do those of most other students of health and social care (Gellis et al, 2003; Bagri and Tiberius, 2010; Wang and Chonody, 2013; Meiboom et al, 2015), with the result that fewer professionals choose to work in this field. Rather less research has been conducted into the attitudes and experiences of the unqualified, unprofessionalised care workforce who provide the bulk of hands-on long-term care (Eymard and Douglas, 2012, p 33). Such research as has been carried out has focused on their status as workers – their poor pay and conditions, their ethnicity, their job turnover and work motivation – rather than their personal experiences of or attitudes toward those to whom they provide care (Howes, 2005, 2008; Montgomery et al, 2005; Banijamali et al, 2014; but see also Stacey, 2005, 2011).

For many such workers, care for frail elderly people is a form of low paid, low status, dirty work, with limited control over the terms and conditions of one's work (Goodridge et al, 1996). Turnover is high, the work demanding, and exposure to body fluids, verbal abuse and physical aggression common (Howes, 2008). Despite feeling ignored and marginalised by the professionals – and at times by the relatives of the person they care for – studies suggest that care workers derive a sense of dignity and worth from their role as carers, because they are the agents of a moral imperative to care that society cannot help but acknowledge (Stacey, 2005). The abjection associated with incapacity does more than corrode the sense of agency of the older infirm person; it risks doing the same for those who care, whose work with frail old people renders them dirty workers. Their work identity is tainted by the same association of abjectness that is attached to infirmity and dependency, of being treated like dirt. What rescues such workers from this position of marginality is their capacity to reframe their work as dignified because it upholds the moral imperative of care, which, however little financial reward it attracts, nevertheless cannot easily be gainsaid by those who evidently care less.

Achieving dignity at work and becoming the effective agent of that imperative frames the person for whom they care as deserving of compassion and pity, but also, necessarily, more helpless, less agentic and much less fortunate than they are. Extracting dignity from work, whether by succeeding in getting a particular difficult task done, establishing a relationship where others have failed, or becoming an emotionally significant figure to those for whom one cares can seem like a zero-sum game, raising oneself up as a carer by getting the better of the people one cares for (Rodriquez, 2011). In contrast to those who call for something to be done, those who have to enact the moral imperative of care are more exposed to what Nietzsche once called 'care's slave morality' (Nietzsche, 1994). In a particularly challenging article, Paley has argued that nursing, by valorising 'caring' at the core of its professional identity, has sought to combat the profession's underlying resentment of its lower status by raising its compassion for vulnerable others to a virtue greater than that displayed by higher status healthcare professions such as those in medicine (Paley, 2002). The result of this, he argues, is that the profession's lower status is confirmed, indulging in a kind of 'philosophical gobbledygook' that avoids ever being judged as 'effective' or 'ineffective' – but just 'good'. How far Paley's critique of nursing can be extended to unprofessionalised groups is difficult to judge, but one could argue that, being even further marginalised in status than other professional groups, including nursing, might well lead to a tendency to extract dignity by practising what Nietzsche termed *'ressentiment'*, 'the unconscious wish to exercise power over others and, by determining their fates, to inflate one's self esteem' (quoted in Paley, 2002, p 31).

Abuse abjection and the dialectic of dependency

Within this nexus of abjection, powerlessness and resentment, abuse becomes an ever present potential occurrence, embedded within the care imperative and its 'slave' morality. The topic of 'elder abuse' appeared first in the professional literature as 'granny bashing', framed as a problem of *families* and informal care (Baker, 1975; Bursto, 1975). Only later was it reformulated as 'elder abuse', and extended to both formal and informal care settings (Eastman, 1984). The initial assumptions that many professionals in the health and social care sector made was that weak or infirm elderly people were abused by younger, fit and healthy adult relatives who felt frustration at the abject plight of their aged dependent parent or partner. Abuse was treated as a reprehensible but understandable reaction to the strain imposed on the fit by the frail.

One of the first researchers to question this assumption was Karl Pillemer. In a study of cases of physical abuse referred to a specialist model programme designed to help older victims of abuse, Pillemer interviewed 42 older people who had suffered physical abuse at the hands of a relative and 42 older people matched in their family circumstances but with no reports of abuse. What Pillemer argued and what his data seemed to show was that the dependency of the *carer* on the *cared for* – whether emotional, financial or practical – was what mostly predicted the presence and extent of elder abuse, not the other way round (Pillemer, 1985). This led to a reappraisal of 'elder abuse' within the family, recognising that it is the inter-dependency or reciprocal dependency between carers and cared for that most fosters abuse. It could be argued that this reflects as much the corrosion of the agency of the carer as that of the person being cared for, and makes it hard for either to escape the unwelcome bonds of their dependency.

Since Pillemer's pioneering research, empirical studies of abuse have proliferated. Recent reviews of this work suggest that (a) abuse usually takes on multiple forms, ranging from verbal to physical abuse, and (b) most abuse is perpetrated by adult children or intimate partners/spouses (Walsh and Yon, 2012). As Manthorpe has noted, so-called carer stress is rarely, on its own, a cause of abuse. The risk for abuse appears to depend more on problematic characteristics associated with the abuser (including their heavy consumption of alcohol or drugs) than it does on any characteristics of the person being abused (Manthorpe, 2015). This reformulation of the nature of abuse, from its presumed reflection of the abject position of the subject of care to that of the agent of care, reinforces our point that it is the mutual abjection of carer and cared for, both of them being immersed in a set of abject circumstances, that creates the conditions for care practices to merge with those of abuse.

What of the abjection of care workers? While most of the research into elder abuse has concentrated on reported cases of 'domestic abuse', abuse within institutions had already been explored from the perspective of the institution and the (mal)practices associated with the total institution (Goffman, 1961). This view of 'institutionalised' abuse meant that less regard was paid to the characteristics of the inmates, patients or residents 'at risk', and more to the systemic features of abuse as 'poor care'. The major distinctions that were highlighted were between (a) impersonal, totalising care and control versus more individualised, person-centred care and (b) high standard, professional care versus low standard, unprofessional care. Abuse arising within the interpersonal relationships between care workers and those for whom they cared for, was, if not totally neglected, consigned to the realm of description rather than analysis (see, for example, Townsend, 1962; Robb, 1967; Vladeck, 1980). Calls for improvements in institutional care – for example, for showing more dignity to patients/residents – generally emphasised the need for systemic improvements and better resources, on the grounds that 'there is a simple and direct relationship between resource levels and dignity, such that the better the resources (money, time, staff, energy, enthusiasm, commitment), the richer the circumstances, the more likely it is that patients will be dignified' (Seedhouse and Gallagher, 2003, p 371). But is institutional abuse so totally different from domestic abuse in either its causes or its manifestations?

To some extent, the answer must be yes. Abuse arising from conflicts, confusion or misunderstandings between residents, for example, is confined entirely to communal settings. Such conflict may be a more common source of abuse than that between staff and residents (Rosen et al, 2008). While abuse taking place between care workers and the people they care for may not seem so obviously distinct from domestic abuse, the care worker is initially a stranger to the person whose often intimate care they provide, and for those with the poorest of memories, they may remain such. It is hardly surprising, then, that abuse towards (and by) care workers occurs most often when cognitively frail residents are receiving intimate care such as that involved in bathing, dressing and washing (Saveman et al, 1999; Zeller et al, 2009; Morgan et al, 2012). These acts of care may appear not as care but as assaults, unwelcomed intimacies and threatening intrusions on the person by relative strangers. It is less clear that abuse and assaults towards, or by, informal carers arise primarily in these kinds of situations at home, although such intimate bodily care may prove at least as difficult as it can be in a residential setting or when performed by paid carers at home.

Although staff who work in long-term care settings are more likely to be the victims of assault and abuse than the residents, staff can be the instigators of abuse. There is insufficient research to determine whether this stems from practices of care, from the characteristics of those they care for, or from the personal competencies of the staff (McDonald et al, 2012). What explanatory research there is suggests that all three factors – the organisation of care, qualities of the care workers and characteristics of the people being cared for – all play a part. Given that a frequent 'trigger' is physical or verbal abuse by residents/care recipients, aggressive responses by staff to such triggers seem to reflect either care workers with personal problems, including drug and alcohol problems, mental health problems and/or family conflicts or a lack of experience or ability to cope, with a consequently lowered tolerance for 'difficulties' presented by residents (Conlie Shaw, 1999; Rabold and Goergen, 2013; Hutchison and Stenfert Kroese, 2015).

Given the low wages, limited opportunities for advancement and the burdensome nature of the 'dirty work' of care – whether stemming from dealing with soiled clothing, bodily fluids or difficult and resistive bodies – what is perhaps surprising is that most of the people who provide care do so without compounding the abjection of residents but with some sense of pleasure or satisfaction within what Rodriquez has termed 'a locally shared moral order' (Rodriquez, 2014, p 152). As part of this moral order, he points out, staff seem to cope with episodes of hostility and aggression by various strategies, one of which he notes involves denying residents agency. Residents' aggression directed toward care workers is reframed as not personal, not meant and consequently no reflection on the quality of their own caregiving. The abjection of both resident and care worker is redeemed by the moral order of care. Abuse, like distaste for other aspects of the job, is kept at bay, and in keeping abuse at bay, the ascription of care as abject is avoided or at least minimised. For those removed from this moral order, distanced observers, the question is often raised – how do these people do this job? Then, when news of abuse in a care home or hospital appears in the media, the question becomes – how could anyone behave so badly toward such poor, vulnerable people? Like a two-sided mirror, the imaginary of the abject class represents the morally pitiable easily reversed as the morally deficient. For those immersed in the nexus of care, the construction of an appropriate narrative order that selectively personalises and depersonalises those receiving care seems necessary in order to avoid confronting a common fate of helpless impotence.

Conclusions

At the beginning of this chapter, we argued that abjection can be seen as a signifier of indigence, a characteristic of persons whose destitution reflects either their impotence or danger. The origins of such abject classes, we would contend, lie in the modern transformation of the economy, in increasing rates of industrialisation and the necessity of selling labour power in order to maintain the individual's household. The inability to work that became a source of private shame increasingly became a cause of public concern, and by the turn of the 20th century, efforts were made to eradicate the abject poverty that had become so associated with age and age-associated impotence. In spite of the success of the post-war welfare state in reducing the absolute poverty that had concerned social reformers like Charles Booth and Seebohm Rowntree, old age remained a category of residual poverty during the immediate post-war decades. With time, however, and with rising wages, improved pension coverage and enhanced welfare benefits, old age ceased to be defined by such a residual status: if not poverty, abject poverty at least seemed to have become a matter of history.

At the turn of the 20th century, the aged and infirm had formed one of the largest groups making up the abject poor. Over the subsequent decades this whole class melted away – a trend that was carefully mapped by Rowntree's studies of the people of York through the first half of the century (Rowntree, 1901, 1941; Rowntree and Lavers, 1951). In its place, and shorn of much of its previous socioeconomic disadvantage, the infirmity of old age – frailty, as it is now called – has emerged to define a new abject class, one almost entirely composed of poor old people defined by their cumulative incapacities and insufficiencies. The abjection of this latter day frailty was reflected in the dependency it represented, leaving it to others to look after the only property that the aged and infirm still possessed, their bodies. As the ageing societies of the post-war period have continued to age, a new divide has become apparent, between those who are 'successfully' ageing – the fit – and those who are not – the frail.

While there were at least some limited options for the old abject classes to perform as social agents, the state of much contemporary old age frailty precludes it. The inability to conceal from others one's abject incapacity is one thing; the unawareness of that incapacity and the consequent failure to experience any desire or need to conceal it is another. Cognitive frailty – dementia – serves to deepen the abjection of corporeal frailty, because it limits the power of the person to either conceal or compensate for their incapacity. Not only do people with dementia lack social agency; they lose the personal agency necessary to 'perform' as other than their attributed status as 'abject'. If there is someone – an informal carer – to share or take on such responsibilities, it may be possible together to shield the frail older person from the full force of such abjection, but as informal care becomes less effective in doing so, the carer's own impotence is revealed. Both carer and cared for risk being irreversibly lost beneath the shadows of the fourth age, and for many, there are no other options than to turn to the 'kindness of strangers'.

Abjection, like frailty, is caught up within the networks of care, and these, in turn, are increasingly caught up with abjection. This nexus of inter-dependency becomes not simply abject, but potentially abusive. The greater the (mental) frailty and the stronger the inter-dependency between carer and cared for, the more insidiously abject and more potentially abusive the relationship becomes. Care, caring relationships and the wider nexus of care that transforms the life world of home into the systems world of the increasingly marketised state cannot be made sense of without some conception of frailty and abjection. But these two concepts alone are not the only conditions that realise care. Such considerations lead us to examine, in the final section of the book, the social relations of care, both as reproductive labour and as moral imperative, its role in sustaining and subverting agency and identity, and thereby in realising and resisting the social imaginary of the fourth age.

SIX

The moral imperative of care

We began this book by outlining our formulation of the fourth age as the cultural reconfiguration of all those aspects of old age that are most associated with fear and disgust. Such a social imaginary, we argued, draws on past and present representations of age as frailty, abjection and loss. The feared loss of agency, identity and independence that constitutes a pervasive element of this social imaginary is now centred on age-associated mental decline linked to 'Alzheimer's disease' (Cutler, 2015). To provide a fuller context to the representation of this anticipated 'loss' within the fourth age's social imaginary, we reviewed how concepts such as agency, identity, and the all-embracing category of 'personhood' have been understood in philosophy and in the social sciences. This overview led us to reconsider the utility of the term 'personhood', both as a way of understanding the losses and limitations that age and infirmity can bring, and as a structure by which the practices of caring for infirm older people are oriented.

We then explored the idea of frailty. We argued that frailty operates as an indicator of both actual and anticipated losses, of present disabilities and future vulnerabilities. Linked to this, the narratives of frailty serve as dividing practices, establishing a social distinction between the fit and the frail, between the senior citizen and the long-term care client. While claims of 'personhood' have sought to establish a communality of ageing based on the notion of a shared vulnerability existing between the already frail and those not yet frail, the construct and use of frailty as a dividing practice has undermined the very possibilities of communality through its association with the rationing of care and services, as well as by the consequent exclusion of the frail. The agentic status of disabled older people is consequently compromised by the extent of their frailty, the depth of their dependency and the institutional responses that result. Claims of personhood, we argued, offer no more protection than has the consumerist approach to care promoted in the last decades of the 20th century (Gilleard and Higgs, 1998). What is needed is a re-examination of care, its meanings and its practices, as well as an examination of the way these narratives and practices compensate for or further constrain the limitations faced by infirm older people in their exercise of agency, the realisation of their capabilities and the expression of their identities.

Turning to the topic of care in this final section, we aim to re-examine its meanings, its moral identity and the relations by which care is socially realised. We accept from the outset the Janus-like role that care of frail older people performs in enabling their lives to be better lived, while also recognising the constraints created in making such 'betterment' possible. Care establishes an identity as it 'takes care' while it takes identity away as it 'gives care'. In and through care the fourth age imaginary is socially realised as both narrative and as practice; it is realised through that which is guarded against and through that which is acknowledged within these practices and narratives. To explore this paradox at the centre of care, we begin by considering care in the abstract, as both a set of narratives, practices and relationships as well as a particular moral imperative, a virtue or ethos.

The nature of care and caring

The last half century has seen a steady growth of interest in care and caregiving. Although it is hard to point to a definite moment of take-off, the topic of 'care' appears to have registered on the academic professional and political agenda sometime in the 1970s, during the first 'crisis' of the post-war welfare state, when the sustainability of state-supported systems of care began to be questioned (Leira, 1994). Concerns over growing demands on the community to look after sick, disabled, frail and vulnerable persons appeared with increasing regularity in the media, in political rhetoric and in the academic and practitioner journals of researchers, clinicians and social care practitioners during the late 1970s and early 1980s. The main emphasis of such concerns was less on defining the nature of care than on determining its limits. How much care could people, the community, family systems tolerate before the stress of caring got 'too much'? Writing in 1989, one of the pioneers of research into the stresses of people caring for frail older relatives, Steven Zarit, gave witness to the 'phenomenal' growth of interest in family caregiving during the preceding decade, when he wondered whether some limit might not soon be reached in funding further research in this area (Zarit, 1989, p 147). No such limits were observed, and the research literature on carer stress and burden continued unabated (Parker, 1990; Twigg, 1992; Cummins, 2001; Ablitt et al, 2009; Schoenmakers et al, 2010).

Following this interest in family care, the concept of 'caregiver burden' and the limits of care came a new focus on defining what was meant by care and what distinguished it from other forms of work or other kinds of relationship. Nel Noddings' book, *Caring: A feminine approach to ethics and moral education*, exemplified this new framework, expanding concern from the difficulties of looking after dependent, frail and ill clients, patients or relatives to the virtues of caring itself – to what might be called its moral identity (Noddings, 1984). Noddings was herself influenced by the work of Carole Gilligan, whose book, *In a different voice*, challenged the masculinist assumptions underpinning theories of moral development and the dominance of Kantian models of morality that paid scant attention to the significance of relationships in constituting moral principles and moral judgements (Gilligan, 1982).

For Noddings, care was an example of a 'feminine' ethic, distinct from the formal principles of moral philosophy exemplified by Aristotle, Hume or Kant. Instead of following their search for abstract principles that would be applicable, irrespective of people's particular circumstances, Noddings argued for the privileging of empathy, of feeling with, and of being 'engrossed' by, the (cared for) other (Noddings, 1984, p 33). Although her work focused mostly on the care exemplified in care work, it has been followed by others who shared in the perspective of care as a generalised ethos that extends beyond particular human relationships to humans' relationships with the world at large (Fisher and Tronto, 1990; Bubeck, 1995; Hrdy, 1999; Kittay, 1999; Nussbaum, 2000; Halwani, 2003).

In a review of the various conceptualisations of care employed in ethical theory, Veatch has distinguished two principal approaches, one treating care as a distinct virtue of the carer, the other treating it as a form of right action (Veatch, 1998). While the latter implies that care is a principle of good behaviour, pre-existing any particular relationship, the former implies that care – or 'caring' – is, like courage, loyalty, love and tenderness, a virtuous manner of being and behaving. Veatch pointed out that some writers have argued that care is more than a principle of right action or of virtue, and applies to the quality of relationships rather than simply to individual persons or actions (Veatch, 1998, pp 220-1). Under such circumstances, Veatch argued, relationships, not persons, embody care, although care, it can be argued, also and necessarily embodies people – both as potential caregivers and potential care recipients.

Related to, but distinguishable from, a concern with 'care ethics' has been a line of sociological research examining care as work – as paid or unpaid labour (Thomas, 1993; Leira, 1994; Himmelweit, 1999; Nelson, 1999; England, 2005). Within this research tradition, care is treated as neither a virtue nor a necessary burden, but as a form of 'reproductive' labour. Within this framework, reproductive labour refers to all those activities and attitudes, behaviours and emotions, responsibilities and relationships directly involved in the maintenance of life on a daily basis, and intergenerationally (Laslett and Brenner, 1989, p 382). From this perspective, care, whether paid or unpaid, is seen as predominantly 'women's work', a role requirement constitutive of a gender rather than a common task or shared human virtue, one modelled on the traditional division of labour within the family (Finch and Groves, 1983). This view of care as a gendered practice is used to explain why paid care work is consistently socially and economically undervalued. In her review of theory and research into care work, England notes that care work has been understood in several potentially different ways, sometimes viewed as low-paid, gendered labour, sometimes as an important but under-acknowledged form of public service, associated with but not confined to 'women's work', and sometimes as work carried out where the intrinsic motivation to care (the moral imperative) competes with and potentially reduces the value of care that is performed for the material rewards of pay and/or status (England, 2005). We shall address these various aspects of care work more fully in the next chapter.

Despite much recent research into the nature of care, Engster has argued that care remains conceptually 'underdeveloped', as does our understanding of the moral imperative to care (Engster, 2005, p 50). Drawing particularly on the work of Tronto (1993), Nussbaum (2000) and Okin (2003/04), Engster distinguishes between the aims of care and the virtues through which it is delivered. Three aims are basic to the practice of care: *helping others* satisfy 'the basic biological needs necessary for survival', *helping others* develop or sustain 'as much as they are able' the capabilities necessary to function as a member of society and pursue their conception of a good life, and finally, *helping others* avoid or have ameliorated pain and suffering in order to better meet their needs and realise their capabilities (Engster, 2005, pp 51-3). Caring involves satisfying these basic aims, 'in a caring way', that is, through the 'virtues of caring'. Following Noddings and Tronto, Engster identifies these as 'attentiveness', 'responsiveness' and 'respect' that are undertaken; what these virtues mean is that care is given to the other much in the way that one cares for oneself. Finally, one other defining and necessary feature to distinguish care from other similar activities is that acts of caring can only be deemed caring if they are designed to meet a need that cannot be met by the person receiving care (Engster, 2005, p 56). 'Servicing' a client – for example, by cutting their hair, serving them dinner or helping them dress – is not care if the person could do this him or herself; cutting someone's toenails or feeding them because they are not able to do these things themselves, on the other hand, is care. So, care cannot be understood either by the aim or the task, or the manner in which (however carefully) an individual performs that task; it has to be framed by the context of the relationship, a distinct, social relationship between a carer who can and a cared-for person who cannot meet their own needs.

Care as a moral or social imperative

While the manner in which care is provided might be considered a reflection of the traits of the carer – their attentiveness, responsivity or respectfulness toward the person they are looking after – whether the imperative to care is a virtue that characterises the moral status of the carer or an imperative that is endemic to society is less clear. From a Kantian perspective, categorical moral imperatives flow from the abstract personhood all individuals, as individuals, possess; it does not arise from the particular traits, social bonds or cultural values of a particular relationship. At its most minimal, the moral imperative to care is dependent on there being a person in need of help and another in a position to help. To use an example from drama – when Pozzo and his servant, Lucky, lay helpless on the ground, in Act Two of Samuel Beckett's *Waiting for Godot*, Vladimir expresses this principle when he calls on his friend Estragon to do something for these stricken figures:

> Let us not waste our time in idle discourse! Let us do something, while we have the chance! It is not everyday that we are needed. Not indeed that we personally are needed. Others would meet the case equally well, if not better. To all mankind they were addressed, those cries for help still ringing in our ears! But at this place, at this moment, all mankind is us, whether we like it or not. (Beckett, *Waiting for Godot*, 2006, p 74)

While society determines that care happens, it is proximity that largely determines who cares for whom. Families care for each other most, because they are at hand. They see the need and heed the call of infants, children, the sick and the frail because they are there, in the household. The imperative of care is realised through such spatial and relational proximity. Who is more likely to notice and respond to another's need for help if not the person closest to them? It is only when the need is so great, or the capabilities to respond so limited, that the call for help stretches beyond the home, evoking responses from neighbours or from the wider community. In short, while the imperative of care might be thought a Kantian requirement of humankind, it is also a necessary response of those closest to the person in need. Only when that imperative cannot be exercised by those close by, those in or close to the household of the person in need, is there a public cry for help, which, emerging as a public cry, becomes a public problem, one that also signifies the 'impotence' of the household from which it rises and the generalised necessity that 'something must be done'.

Made public, the imperative to do something comes with the possibility of shame, shame that may be experienced by all the persons in the household, to the extent that they, as autonomous rational agents, have failed to help and risk bringing shame on the community to the extent that it, too, fails to be up to the task of helping. While it can be argued that this sort of argument fails to address the gendered nature by which these imperatives to care are realised within the household, it serves to illustrate how, in the transition in the locus of care from the domestic to the public realm, while the inability to provide care becomes a source of shame, the person judged 'uncared for' becomes a subject of abjection. While informal care is now framed as part of the public realm, thereby confounding the salience of this transition (and arguably making care of all sorts more similar to work and its exchange a function of markets), the abjection brought about by the inadequacy of care depends on it being publicly perceived as such, not on any inherent property of the care recipient or on the nature of his or her particular impairments.

The necessity of doing something about the particular weaknesses or incapacities that elicit care, as well as the criteria of adequacy in meeting those responsibilities, have varied over time and across communities. While moral philosophy has existed for centuries, and the precept to help those in need has probably been in existence even longer, the way that care is provided outside the individual household has not obviously derived from any particular, constant ethos of care, that is, one that specifies the who and the what, if not exactly the that, of care. Variations in the sense of responsibilities of care between and within households as well as variations in the practices that are deemed to constitute 'help' or the circumstances that constitute 'need' reflect differences in the structure of households and communities and in the resources available in particular societies at particular times.

Reher (1998), for example, has argued that historical differences in household forms between Northern and Southern Europe led to marked regional differences in the social relations of care. The Southern model encourages inter-generational proximity for much longer than the Northern model, and holds the generalised expectation that in times of difficulty, family should be the first and often only port of call for help. In such societies, Reher quotes a Spanish saying, that 'the only really poor person is one who has no family' (Reher, 1998, p 212). Consequently, he argues, civil society has been weaker in Southern Europe, where systematic community provision for the poor and the vulnerable has been lacking or has been made available in relatively unsystematic forms, reflecting the significance of the almsgiving rather than any considered civic or communal appraisal of public need. He contrasts this Southern model with the more extensive set of formal communal provision observed in Northern Europe, especially after the Reformation, when the late medieval pattern of largely uncontrolled and unregulated charitable giving concentrated within the major cities was replaced by more comprehensive networks of organised care.

Reher goes on to speculate that even the 'strong' families of Mediterranean society are only 'relatively' strong, when compared with, for example, 'the strict allegiances and corporatism generated within enlarged family lineages and clans that characterize large regions of Asia' (Reher, 1998, p 215). While it is beyond the scope of this book to pursue in the necessary detail the precise moral framework and social relations of care that operate in non-Western societies, it is worth recognising that even within the confined geography of Western Europe, profound historical and geographical differences have existed in the organisation and meaning attached to providing care outside the family, and by implication, the 'distributional' norms of care, and, one might add, the consequent 'strength' of the shame that is attached to any publicly recorded expression of household helplessness and kinship insufficiency.

It is a matter of conjecture that variations in the shame attached to such impotence might be dependent on the balance between the domestic and civic sources of social capital. Societies with large close-knit families and fewer and weaker civic institutions might be thought to bring down more shame to households and kin in failing to look after their members than in societies with less domestic but more civic social capital. This does not mean that the care given within such households is of a higher quality, or more extensive or more lovingly given; it could well be the opposite, as families refusing outside help strive inadequately to care for those with the greatest vulnerability. Likewise one might predict that where there is less shame attached to the evident impotence of households to look after their own, there may be higher expectations from civic institutions to meet the needs of care, since the 'entitlement' to care and support from these institutions would be correspondingly greater. In short, even if care may be considered an abstract moral imperative (in the sense of an imperative to help those who are unable to help themselves), its particular nature, meaning and the virtues by which it is delivered will be contingent on a wider set of expectations, norms and values. This is perhaps what Thomas meant when she wrote that care 'is an empirical category, not a theoretical one', whose forms 'remain to be theorised in terms of other theoretical categories' (Thomas, 1993, p 668). From this kind of perspective, we cannot avoid dealing with issues of theoretical importance that shape the relations of care, including those of 'agency', 'identity', 'self' and 'other'; our preference, however, is to treat these, as much as possible, as sociological rather than moral or metaphysical phenomena.

The social relations of care: formal and informal care

When we speak of the social relations of care we are alluding to two related but distinct forms of care. Just as one can distinguish between the realm of domestic production and its social relations and production for the market – whether through selling one's labour power or selling the products of one's labour – so it is possible to distinguish between the social relations of care within the family (informal care) and the social relations of care within the community (formal care). Just as domestic production cannot be understood without reference to the wider operations of the market, so 'informal' care provided within the family cannot be understood without reference to the organisation of care existing outside of it in the wider community. The boundaries between formal and informal social relations of care are relative as are the features distinguishing between the two; the social imaginary of the fourth age neither begins nor ends at the threshold of home.

Nevertheless, distinctions can be made that have particular relevance to how ideas of agency and identity are interwoven in areas of practice such as dementia care. Formal as well as informal care are not equal sources of the social imaginary of a fourth age, and nor are they equal sources of protection against it. We discuss formal care work in more detail in the next chapter. In the rest of this chapter, we outline our case for maintaining and using this admittedly problematic division. Broadly speaking, care given and received within the household by those within the household constitutes the prototype for the relations of care and its idealisation as a moral or social imperative. Care provided from outside the household attracts a social and usually financial cost to the householder, thereby rendering it subject to a more explicitly economic framework that is closer to the purchasing of services than it is to the exchange of affection and support expected in families and within the household. While informal care evolves out of closeness and affinity, formal care begins with a negotiated distance. The social relations of care and care work can be further distinguished from those of service relationships, since all forms of care hinge on the assumption that the person receiving care is incapable of performing the tasks that the carer performs on his or her behalf. If the person receiving assistance is deemed capable of doing the task him- or herself, then doing what the person can do for him- or herself is rendering them a service; it is not care.

This distinction between providing informal or formal care and providing a service also embodies differences in power and status. Care providers have greater agency and status than care recipients; this is the opposite for service work, when the service providers have less. Although treating formal care as a paid service can seem to confound these distinctions, informal care, if and when performed without reference to formal care, does not. The carer possesses more agency and status whether or not he or she receives any form of payment, and however much the service provider is paid, his or her status can never trump that of the person who purchases their services. The ambiguities of informal care lie in the gradual and often imperceptible transformation of one kind of relationship (parent–child, husband–wife, etc) into another; such ambiguities do not affect formal care since the carer arrives in that role, as a stranger. In this latter case, the ambiguities in formal care arise in the indistinct boundary between control and capability, and the agentic status of the care or service recipient. Are they 'really' in need, incapable, or are they 'really' treating the carer like a 'servant' and 'the home' as if it were 'a hotel'?

Within such ambiguities of care, issues of identity, agency and power are played out. While the carer can easily be understood as someone doing something for some other individual who cannot, it would be a mistake to assume that the latter's identity and power are erased as a result. Even if agency is not a necessary attribute of the care recipient, identity is, and with identity come issues of status and power. The care recipient may be asleep, unconscious, or even in a coma while the carer washes, watches over or carries out tasks for him/her, but their identity to the carer may remain that of a much loved mother, uncaring partner or soul mate. While these identities do not necessarily confer agency on the care recipient, they may nevertheless influence what, how much, and in what ways informal care and help are given. In the case of formal care delivered by a stranger to a disabled older person, not only is the extent of the care recipient's agency constrained by providing such care as 'care work' rather than a 'service', but so, too, is the range of identities elicited by such care work. Arguably, the phenomenon of 'social death' often associated with illness and infirmity in old age reflects not so much to a lack of agency as a lack of social identity (Mulkay, 1992; Gilleard and Higgs, 2015).

Identity, agency and ambiguity in informal care

Like formal care work, informal care possesses its own ambiguities. These, too, are associated with issues of agency and identity. Not only does the moral identity of family members vary during the processes of negotiating care, but so, too, does that of the care relationship itself (Finch and Groves, 1983). Relationships between spouses or partners may be viewed – or valued – more for their affective than for their instrumental value, and the instrumental services performed (bringing in money, making meals, organising holidays, taking children to school, washing and ironing clothes, etc) may be valued as signs of love or affection, or indicators of valued personal qualities in one's partner, such as kindness or thoughtfulness, rather than as indicators of instrumental assistance and of labour performed. It may not matter that a husband, for example, is able to cook, clean or wash; his wife may perform these services for them both, out of feelings of love, or because their performance reinforces her identity as a 'loving wife and mother'. This does not mean that one or other partner may not at times perceive their role within the household as 'work' and complain that they are being treated as a 'skivvy', or a 'handyman', or even as 'a walking wallet'. But such possible identities exist to be called on at particular times and circumstances – minor narratives, as it were, that are capable, especially if and when affection declines, to becoming more salient, dominant discourses. When the husband or wife loses his or her ability to perform various household tasks ('instrumental activities of daily living', in the terminology of gerontological research), and the partner takes over (or continues), the point of transition from 'care' given as expressed affection to 'care' given as necessary assistance may be harder to identify when the affectional relationship is retained – when a couple still love each other and these other identities and their supporting narratives remain salient. On the other hand, when 'care' as affection for the other has long gone, or was never much developed, and the relationship serves primarily to maintain the household and with it the couple's identities, this transition may be realised more clearly and perhaps more bitterly (Adams, 2006).

Other transitions to informal care may be easier and less painful to identify, as when an adult child recognises the gradual loss of capabilities in his or her parent. Here, the affectional bond between child and parent will already have undergone a number of transformations much before any decline in a parent's capabilities, for example, as adult children leave home and establish separate households and social networks. Parental power, and, to some extent, love for the parent, usually lessens as partnering and being partnered replace parenting and being parented, and the family of origin no longer serves as 'home' (Swartz, 2009; Silverstein and Giarrusso, 2010).

This distancing of attachment and identity may give adult children a more 'objective' view of their parents and a greater likelihood of noticing changes in their parents' capabilities, character and concerns. Even so, a preparedness to acknowledge loss or decline in one's parents' competence, power and status is often qualified by the continuing value that a mother or father may have to the sense of identity of their adult children. Parents, however frail, can serve as a kind of shield protecting their children from fully acknowledging the consequences of their adulthood and its intimations of mortality. Acknowledging or denying any weakness in that shield may, for some adult children, for some time, affect how they attend and respond to their parent's mental or physical infirmity. The shadows of the fourth age may be kept at bay by partners or children who refuse to relinquish their other older identities or concede any loss of identity or power in the other. By refusing to have to care or label what one does as care, the other escapes being rendered dependent and 'other' and their relationship redefined (Gaugler et al, 2003). Of course, if and when such implicit strategies are undermined – for whatever reason – the loss is irretrievable, and the shadows of the fourth age loom larger (Førsund et al, 2015).

The renegotiations of identities and relationships involve not just the 'carer to be' but also the person 'to be cared for'. Older people who develop impairments and infirmities differ in their own recognition of these weaknesses, some of which may be harder to detect or acknowledge than others. The father who has had a stroke, the mother who has developed osteoarthritis, the husband who has become diabetic, or the wife who is suffering from early dementia are each in line for becoming 'dependents' in different ways and at different rates. But aside from the determinacy of the conditions creating dependency, the older person him- or herself is also a potential agent in that process. It is as agents that they, too, contribute to constructing – or resisting – care. While the overwhelming focus of the research literature on later life infirmity and 'informal' caregiving has been on the actions, experiences and subjectivity of the caregiver(s), the agency and identity of the potential care recipient has been neglected, as has their role in helping shape and in turn being shaped by care (Wiles, 2011, p 576). It is to this 'co-construction' of care and agency between the carer and the cared to which we now turn.

Agency in the co-construction of care

Even the most helpless of people exercise some degree of agency in the care relationship despite the disparities in health and social capital that may exist between them and their carer(s). The way such agency is or is not represented plays a crucial role in realising or resisting the fourth age social imaginary. The process whereby any (informal) caring relationship is established, the transitions that mark its 'career' and the potential for it to bring about its own abjection can be understood in both agentic and structural terms – such that one may focus on only one agent, typically the carer, or on disability and infirmity as the corporeal 'actant', or on the pre-existing classed, gendered and kinship relationship. To date, we would argue, academic and professional emphases have privileged the former two – coping with care and the effects of infirmity (often named as in Alzheimer's, cancer, Parkinson's or stroke). There has been less consideration given to the co-construction of care (Graham and Bassett, 2006; Davies, 2011).

Once infirmity has created multiple needs for help, the person being cared for still retains a degree of agency within the care relationship, although this is rarely greater or equal to that of their carer(s). By way of illustration, a person who is quite old and infirm may still reciprocate in the practices of care. They can actively facilitate care, for example, by lifting up an arm so that the carer can wash underarms, or by linking arms when the carer and cared for take a walk. Equally and oppositely, it is possible for the person being cared for to demonstrate negative agency by actively refusing to be cared for. The individual living alone may refuse to let the carer into his or her house; he or she may refuse to get undressed for the planned bath, or resist being taken to the toilet after soiling or wetting the bed. Resistance or refusal to be cared for may be no less a reflection of agency as active acquiescence in care, but it is more problematic because it confounds the possibility for the carer to perform as a carer despite the incapacities of the person designated as 'needing help'. These struggles over agency and identity can be represented in different ways – as a reflection of character (for example, 's/he's being bloody minded/obstinate/stupid', etc) or of impairment (lack of insight, failure of understanding), but the carer more often than not is the person with the power to frame the narrative to others, if not to insist on its truth value to the person being cared for. The choice of narrative – of lost agency or changed identity compared with changed agency and lost identity – presents a further problem for care, in that it risks undermining the moral identity of both carer and cared for, as well as compromising that of their relationship (for example, as between two adults equally close to each other).

Care relationships are dynamic. For much of the time, caring rarely represents a fixed status or a fixed identity. Positions may be held firmly and certain identities made salient one day while being overshadowed by other concerns the next day. One day the carer may not feel like washing under the person's arms; one day the person cared for may not want to link arms and go for a walk; one day the person receiving care may express immense gratitude, another day little or none. The agency of carer and cared for remains fluid even after the roles of carer and cared for are more or less accepted, and it would be a mistake to imply that care completely transforms a person's identity or necessarily restricts their agency, such that every frail older person who lives with and is looked after by family or friends is thereby consigned to a fourth age imaginary or is treated as if they were socially 'dead' (Sweeting and Gilhooly, 1997; Gilleard and Higgs, 2015). Care need not cease even if it is no longer co-constructed in the way it once was; loss of agency need not mean loss of identity. Mutuality between carer and cared for can be maintained with a minimum of 'passive' agency for a considerable time, and care relationships can hold, even when agency does not.

Reciprocity and the care relationship

Although the play of agency, identity and power in the care relationship depends on the players, rarely do they remain of equal strength. Sometimes, it is true, an elderly couple will say, "He is my eyes, I am his memory", and together manage to support and care for each other's complementary weaknesses, with a sense of shared agency and identity. Such symmetry is, however, not so common; in most cases, the carer comes to exercise greater agency over a wider domain of domestic life than the person he or she is caring for. But even as changes in power and role take place within the relationship, these changes need not bring down the shadows of a fourth age. One major factor in safeguarding the relationship from the fourth age imaginary is the continuing reciprocity of the relationship, even if it is rarely as complete as the above example suggests.

In the large body of research that has been conducted over the last few decades into the degree of 'burden' felt by carers looking after an older infirm family member, reciprocity has been shown consistently to protect the relationship from break down and/or excessive burden (Horowitz and Shindelman, 1983; Morris et al, 1988; Dwyer et al, 1994; Carruth et al, 1997; Reid et al, 2005; Graham and Bassett, 2006; Del-Pino-Casado et al, 2014). Although most research has focused on the effects of reciprocity on carers' feelings of burden or stress, studies focusing on care recipients have shown the importance that reciprocity has for the wellbeing of people receiving care (Wolff and Agree, 2004). The meaning of reciprocity, however, has not always been critically examined. The distinction between reciprocity as generalised social exchange common to most social relations (Dowd, 1975; Cook, 1987) and reciprocity as a distinct form of mutuality that is confined to close or intimate relationships (Hirschfeld, 1983) is often overlooked. When reciprocity is framed as part of the general give-and-take of social relationships, it has been claimed that frailty or infirmity prevents equal exchange, in effect, blocking reciprocity (Gouldner, 1973). Others have suggested that despite such circumstances, reciprocity can be maintained, but only at the expense of the care recipient 'ceding' power to the carer (Dowd, 1975, 1980). Equating reciprocity with mutuality, Hirschfeld has argued that carers continue to find gratification in their relationship with the person they care for, either out of their own sense of love, gratitude and identity attributed to the past and present relationship, or from the evident affection, closeness and gratitude that is still displayed by the person being cared for (Hirschfeld, 1983). Although she has introduced the concept within the context of informal or family care, where the relationship draws on past as well as present affectional bonds and mutual exchange, others have sought to extend it to 'care work' relationships (Henson, 1997). We discuss the relevance of mutuality and reciprocity in care work relationships in the next chapter.

Others have argued that reciprocity in the care relationship is multi-dimensional, and that when asked about their understanding of their relationship with the care recipient, family carers of infirm older relatives used the term in different ways. In one Danish study, Lewinter found that there was recognition of a generalised reciprocity – returning current caregiving for the care he or she had received in the past from their relative – as well as the specific reciprocity of affection felt and gratitude received (Lewinter, 2003, p 372). Achieving mutuality and an appropriate balance between care given and gratitude received is difficult enough even in the everyday relationships between partners or parents and their adult children; the differential vulnerability of the carer and the care recipient make balance and mutuality much harder to realise with any degree of constancy. If achieved, the protective value seems indubitable. In one prospective study of people with dementia and their (informal) carers, Norton and her colleagues were able to demonstrate that close relationships, especially between husbands and wives, resulted in significantly slower rates of mental and functional decline over a two-year period (Norton et al, 2009). Likewise, the willingness to continue to care, resistance to the idea of institutionalising one's partner or parent and the refusal to consider the person being cared for as 'socially dead' seem, in part, at least, dependent on a sense of mutuality and feelings of reciprocity (Sweeting and Gilhooly, 1997; Wells, 1999; Heru and Ryan, 2006; Brodaty and Donkin, 2009).

Set against these protective factors is the progressive strain faced by those who care, increasing in intensity as the person being cared for becomes less aware of their own and their carers' difficulties – making living with and caring for someone with dementia more difficult than most other chronic medical conditions (Brodaty and Donkin, 2009). At some point it can seem as if the choice is no longer about the degree of mutuality that can be sustained between them, but rather the risk that both will become forever lost under the darkening shadows of the fourth age. The more agentic partner eventually faces baling out as much as an act of self-preservation as a rejection of their role as carer. The reasons for such decisions are complex, involving as they do considerations of their limited capabilities, the care recipient's incapacities, each person's health as well as a variety of other factors affecting the viability of the household (Afram et al, 2014). But whatever reasons may be given – to themselves, to others (including researchers into care) – there are few who in making or being made to accede to such decisions escape the consequent sense of guilt and shame that this may bring, the feeling one has failed to care enough. Informal care has its invisible limits.

Care and its corporeal constraints

While mutuality within the care relationship plays an important role in constructing and maintaining it, given the fact that most people with dementia spend their final months – or years – in a nursing or residential home (Houttekier et al, 2010), other factors beyond the care relationship come to exercise a more powerful influence. Transferring the care recipient and much of their care to the agency of strangers runs the risk of bringing down the shadows of the fourth age, even as it prevents the carer's own self and identity from being erased. While informal care rarely ceases after a person is admitted to a nursing or residential care facility, as the bed and the person are transferred to the care of strangers, care becomes more obviously more one-sidedly 'care work', and the social imaginary of the fourth age comes closer to enveloping the person entering a 'new' and 'strange' home from home. While many aspects of that imaginary could be ignored or denied, before, during and after the transition from kinship to informal care, with the transition to formal care they cannot.

In the context of familiar, informal care, the person being cared for need not actively assert their agency and identity since their identity and interests can be easily accepted, trading on past habits and shared identities. Removed from that context, new demands are called for at the point at which, ironically, they are least likely to be met. Within the new community of co-residents and carers only an abstract residency-citizenship will be granted the newcomer, this often occurring without any articulation of identity or expression of agency. In these circumstances the particularities of their incapacities and their acquiescence (or indeed, their resistance to being helped) will assign them their new, 'residualised' identity. How else can they be known as particular people with narrative identities given that these can no longer be consistently or coherently expressed? What memories they have are lodged and articulated elsewhere, in past selves, past relationships, accessible only as biography.

Not everyone entering a nursing home or residential home will do so because they are suffering from dementia. Frailty and institutionalisation have other causes that may well permit older people to continue to express past and present identities and perform as agentic persons, negotiating and co-constructing their care, even in the context of a nursing home and with care delivered by strangers. Care is not just a function of unequally matched agents possessing or developing moral identities in the context of varying degrees of mutuality. Its activation of particular identities and engagement within the relationship varies with the type and degree of disability and impairment. But most people entering long-term care facilities, particularly nursing homes, do so with some degree of mental infirmity, if not a diagnosis of dementia. Slow shifts in agency and identity may occur, during the course of their stay, especially if the care recipient becomes progressively less able to articulate and express their subjectivity. Inevitably, this leaves the other carers to take on progressively greater responsibility for the kind, style and quality of the relationship. As infirmity, of whatever nature, increases, the agency and identity of the person being cared for becomes less easily expressed. Gradually it is reshaped by the narratives of others, including those 'outside' the informal care relationship

(O'Connor, 2007). The extent to which the shadows of the fourth age darken not just over the person but over the care relationship reflect the degree to which both person and relationship become defined by others, identities to be acquiesced with or resisted, but unlikely ever to be supplanted by the agency and identity of the person being cared for. Formal care for older infirm persons appears to be a 'zero-sum' game, particularly as it is represented by older people entering a home suffering from dementia.

To what extent does this constitute a paradigm for all 'elder' care? Research has shown repeatedly that dementia is more feared than any other age-related condition, that it is a source of greater and more progressive disablement, and provides the most common 'medical' reason for admission into long-term care facilities (Martikainen et al, 2009; Luppa et al, 2010b; Hung et al, 2012; Cutler, 2015). Alzheimer's has come to be feared precisely because it seems to take away agency and identity, leaving the body an orphan in search of a home. Although there is growing recognition that the diagnosis of Alzheimer's does not, in and of itself, deny the possibility of agency and narrative identity – witness the growing number of autobiographical accounts of living with the condition (de Boer et al, 2007; Rodriquez, 2013) – the neuro-degeneration underlying this diagnosis leads sooner or later toward an advanced state of mental and physical decay (unless death intervenes), which is accompanied by institutionalisation and increasingly distressing symptoms and burdensome interventions (Mitchell et al, 2009; Houttekier et al, 2010). There is little evidence that the trajectory of deterioration in mental function and self-care ability is much influenced by macro-aspects of social structure such as class, gender or social capital (Grill et al, 2014; Staff et al, 2016), although much the same may be said of most clinical interventions (Sink et al, 2005; Tschanz et al, 2011; Sona et al, 2012).

Longitudinal studies point to enormous variability in the age of onset and rate of progress of mental deterioration in dementia as well as the appearance, evolution and disappearance of various behavioural or psychiatric problems that can make living with dementia for some, for some time, a dreadful and undignified experience. Given the uncertainty, the mixture of same self and lost self as well as the confusions of agency, the nature of the journey, if not the destination, remains unpredictable and seemingly idiosyncratic. Such uncertainties provide almost as many reasons for optimistic as opposed to pessimistic narratives, and support innumerably different readings of the links between dementia and personhood along the path of this journey. But how far do other conditions create alternative readings of care and its various narratives and practices? Just as developmental difficulties conceal a world of difference beyond that envisioned by the narrow field of severe mental handicap, so the corporeal varieties of later life illness and infirmity cannot all be reflected within the darkening mirror of dementia.

Bodies can fail on their own. A range of chronic conditions affect people with increasing frequency as they grow older. Some cause greater difficulties in self-care and household maintenance than others, but all can be thought of as reducing the reserves of the older person. Broadly speaking, one can think of the variety of illnesses and infirmities of later life as causes of disability, of distress, of decline, and of death. Some, such as stroke, encompass all four; others, such as arthritis, are associated with the first but not the last two. Some, like many cancers, cause death but with only limited or very brief periods of disability or decline; while others, such as depression, lead to unending distress without obvious disability or decline. Given that most of these conditions increase in prevalence with age, it is obvious that the older the person, the more likely he or she will be to acquire multiple morbidities and face disablement, distress, decline and death arising from multiple causes. This is, in essence, the rationale for old age medicine.

To what extent are there differences in the nature and form of care provided to people without dementia but with other chronic illnesses, and how might such differences affect the care relationship? There is less research on family carers of older people with other chronic illnesses compared with the vast literature on care for people with Alzheimer's disease, cognitive impairment or dementia. What there is suggests that 'caregiver resources, not patient diagnosis or illness severity, are the primary predictors of facets of caregiver burden and other caregiver outcomes' (Burton et al, 2011, p 418). There appear to be few signs that the caregiving burden or difficulties increase as these illnesses progress, nor that proximity to death significantly affects the caregiver or the caregiving relationship (Grov and Valeberg, 2012; Sautter et al, 2014). At the risk of over-generalisation, it seems plausible to suggest that affective bonds, the co-construction of care by both carer and cared for, and an evident reciprocity within the relationship sustain most informal care relationships, no matter what aid has to be provided, and no matter how potentially abject the situation may become. The progressive loss of agency and identity that is associated with dementia – and with similar cognitive impairments such as in cases of Parkinson's, stroke or other severe neurological disease – undermines many of the possibilities for the co-construction of care and the maintenance of a shared identity that sustains the relationship. This leads care to become, increasingly, a relationship of one. It is less the weight of corporeal need that overwhelms care and brings down the shadows of the fourth age than the failing mind and the orphaned body it leaves behind.

Conclusions

Care, in the most general sense of helping people in need, is a moral imperative realised in most households. It is less the existence of care that requires explanation than its nature, meanings and the relationships within which it is realised. It is the gendered nature of care, the capacity of households to care, the tasks subsumed under the term 'care', the balance between love and duty in giving care, and the expectations by households that society will supplement or replace their care that invite questions about the care of frail, infirm older people. Care is locked into the life cycle, shaping and being shaped by it. It decreases exponentially in the years following birth, and increases in the years before death.

In this chapter we have distinguished between three facets of care. The first treats care as an ethos, whether as a reflection of right action and the exercise of responsibility that forms part of the social contract or as a moral quality of the person who cares, a virtuous affect. The second treats care as a practice, a set of tasks or obligations – carried out for love and/or money – that is both part of the social exchange within and between households and a core component of modern professions. The third treats care as a relationship emerging out of and transforming other, pre-existing relationships, in the case of informal care, or in the case of formal care, a necessary transaction, a distinct type of contracted-for service where the service provider, not the recipient, possesses more status and holds much of the power (although much of that power may be vested in the service managers rather than the direct providers).

Choosing to pursue this latter model – care as a relationship – in the rest of this chapter, we have focused on the relationships of informal care, particularly those associated with caring for a person with progressive mental infirmity, typically dementia. While we recognise that many people are part of a care relationship involving an older dependent person, who may have little or no mental infirmity, the close relationship between agency, identity and dementia mean that such care is more likely than others to be conducted under the shadow of the fourth age's imaginary. The actual or threatened loss of agency, control and identity that makes dementia more feared than other chronic conditions, presents dilemmas in care that if still present when older care recipients suffer from other chronic conditions, are both more scarcely felt and more easily resisted.

Care for mentally infirm older people risks bringing down closer the shadows of the fourth age as much as it strives to prevent them engulfing the relationship because of the inequality in agency and identity that so often grows between carer and cared for. While mutuality, the co-construction of care, a shared history and intertwined identities can provide a shield, for a time at least, the progressive limitations of the person being cared for reduce the scope for sharing and increase the likelihood that care becomes a relationship of one, that is maintained, repaired and renewed each day more and more by the caring other, and less and less by the person being cared for. This journey through care leads more often than not to the transfer of care practices to another, and typically to someone who is a stranger to what has gone before. What was once a relationship imbricated in past and present concerns is replaced by another sort of care that is now the work of strangers, even if it is done by strangers who mostly labour as much for love as for money.

SEVEN

Care work

In the previous chapter we explored care and its generic realisation in a variety of social relations. Although care can be viewed through the lens of moral philosophy – as a moral duty that is realised through a set of practices embodying distinct virtues – care itself, we argued, can only ever be socially realised within particular forms of relationship. Questions such as who should receive and who should provide care, how and where care should be delivered, and what care means to those who are carers and to those who are cared for will elicit different answers at different times and in different places. Granted this variability in its social forms and relations, it is still the case that an imperative to care remains. There are no societies without care and no care without social proximity – within and between households. Care by those with whom a person lives seems to be a universal reference point for all subsequent social relations of care, whatever form they take and however they are realised. At its simplest, mothers care for their babies, parents care for their children and, when older, their children will care for their partners and eventually for their parents, too.

Within most contemporary care relationships, a central distinction can be made between care given and received by members of a household and care that is provided by others not otherwise related to the person being cared for. This distinction is commonly framed as that between formal/paid and informal/unpaid care. However, it is important to remember that family care seems to still provide the template for other forms of care work, rendering both formal and informal care as forms of reproductive labour. Services provided to families by others can, however, be considered through an alternative or complementary template, representing the social relations of paid care work reflected in the idea of contract and the 'professionalisation' of care (Meagher, 2006). From such a perspective, care services form a distinct part of the market economy, separate from, if not unconnected to, the life-world of family and home. It is this expanding domain of formal care services and the contradictory ways it can be understood that the present chapter addresses.

The relative balance between the two forms of care has undergone a historical shift. Over the last half century care has moved from being predominantly a part of the social relations of the family towards becoming predominantly a service that is paid and provided for from outside the household. This transformation has been variously described as the 'commoditisation of care' (Ungerson, 2002; Green and Lawson, 2011), the 'outsourcing of care' (Bittman et al, 1999; Hondagneu-Sotelo, 2001), or as care's 'defamilialisation' (Esping-Anderson, 1999). Others, however, have rejected this kind of terminology, arguing that it frames this shift in a critical and condemnatory way – as if the former is morally superior to the latter (Folbre and Wright, 2012, p 2). Material and moral considerations arguably play a part in both. What is undoubtedly true is that care and care relationships are being transformed into care work, that is, care given and/or received by paid non-household, non-kin agents (Duffy, 2015).

Various reasons for this change have been proposed. These include the rising level and range of capacities required of both young and old to function in modern societies, which exceed most households' resources; the declining level of domestic social capital, with households becoming smaller and the necessity for adults of childbearing age to be employed outside of the home becoming greater; and finally, rising levels of incapacity and infirmity within households as a function of demographic ageing (the ageing of the old) as well as the increased survival of young people with incapacitating illnesses (Oropesa, 1993; Hochschild, 1999; de Ruijter, 2004). The transition of the mentally frail older person from being located within the network of informal social exchange and care within the family to being a citizen-resident in a formal institutional care facility is especially emblematic of this change.

It is, however, just one expression of a more general transformation. It is perfectly possible to use the outsourcing of childcare or the expansion of domestic labour as examples of the transformation of care equal in their social import. The interpretation of all such transitions is, unsurprisingly, problematic. It could be argued, for example, that expanding care beyond the members of the household benefits both the care recipients and society more generally since formal care is less imbued with a sense of obligation and can be more clearly assessed and its quality publicly judged (Galvin, 2004, p 138). An alternative formulation can represent the transition as the exchange of care within a loving family relationship for more distant objectifying regimes promoted by public institutions or marketised agencies with the risk that such care is inadequately delivered 'out of sight' of those who (should) care. Whatever interpretation is placed on this transition, the rising significance of formal care work cannot be denied. Whether examined as a form of labour (or service), as a set of professionalised practices or as a substitute for or supplement to the social relations of family care, formal care has become the focus of a growing body of research from which this chapter draws (Clarke and Wheeler, 1992; Himmelweit, 1999; Parton, 2003; England, 2005).

In what follows we aim to examine some of the historical continuities and discontinuities of formal care work, its key elements, as realised in care for frail older people, and finally, the narratives that frame the moral identity of such care work, whether as necessary labour or valued professional skill. In doing so, we focus on both care work that is provided to infirm older people in their own home, and that which is provided in formal, institutional settings. We explore its potential both for supplying intimacy and sustaining identity as well as its capacity to undermine agency and invalidate identity; in that sense, we describe its potential to be simultaneously a source of shelter against and a harbinger of the shadows of the fourth age social imaginary. We examine this potential for producing both good and harm as it is realised in the various narratives surrounding formal care provision as well as engaging with its role in shaping and sustaining the identity of care work and care workers, and the various practices that constitute these formal systems of care.

Care work of infirm older people: a brief history

As noted, the lack of available kin and the limited resources of existing kin to provide care to older people first emerged as a serious social problem in the transition from a rural to an industrial economy. It has become a matter of rising concern in post-industrial ageing societies. Before concentrating on an analysis of contemporary care work it is valuable to consider the larger picture in order to set care work within the framework of evolving forms of welfare provision. The idea of a welfare state was based on the recognition that within an industrial society, where the successful reproduction of the household relies on the exchange of labour power, not all households will acquire or possess the resources to meet all the needs and realise all the capabilities of their members (Marshall, 1992). As Sen and others have pointed out, functions, needs and capabilities are not fixed but depend on a given social and cultural context (Sen, 1999). Some functions are more easily realised and some needs more easily met than others; others emerge, evolve and change as society itself changes. In most circumstances, households are expected to be able to meet their material needs, such as food and shelter. Few households possess the resources to educate and train their own children to the point that they can earn their own living and maintain an independent household. Even fewer have the resources to treat illness and injuries or alleviate pain and suffering. That there should be accessible institutions whereby households can meet these needs is a defining feature of 'First Modernity' (Beck et al, 2003), reaching its apogee in the post-war welfare state, during the immediate decades after the Second World War.

Within the British Isles, the *locus classicus* of the industrial revolution, almshouses and asylums, hospitals and hospices, poorhouses and workhouses provided the main infrastructure for meeting such needs, along with orphanages, elementary schools and technical colleges. The multiplication of need and the conjunction of impotence, poverty and sickness contained within these institutions led to a growing sense of public 'shame' at the inadequate way many such institutions were meeting those needs (Himmelfarb, 1991). At the risk of considerable simplification, the impotence of poverty and ignorance were more easily met by the introduction of age and disability pensions, sickness and unemployment pay and universal primary education (Gilleard and Higgs, 2005). Incapacity and impotence arising from disablement and infirmity proved harder to address. Despite the introduction of improved facilities in hospitals for the chronic sick and the more extensive training of doctors and nurses, the numbers of frail and ill older people occupying hospital beds grew. As acute medical care improved and methods of investigation and treatment led to better outcomes, the problems posed by those, typically older patients who failed to respond to the new healthcare regimes, but only accumulated more illnesses and disabilities, proved recalcitrant. For them, the practices of chronic hospital care competed with the mechanisms of 'unblocking beds'.

Care work of infirm older people involves extended periods of what Julia Twigg has referred to as 'body work' (Twigg, 2000; Twigg et al, 2011). Once upon a time, for some well-resourced households, the 'somebody' doing the caring might have been a servant or a maid, and the one being cared for, a master or a mistress. Unlike those who were cared for by such of their kin who were able and available, the person being cared for by a servant would have a certain status. Being in a position to turn care into a service was thus a sign of social power rather than a public display of impotence. Those unable, or unwilling, to perform these tasks, but who could draw neither on kin nor afford servants, would have to rely on receiving their intimate care from their fellow paupers in the workhouse. Within the workhouse infirmaries, the nature of such body work was confined to such ministrations as were provided by fellow paupers, supplemented in the case of Ireland by nuns and sisters who performed their care under the religious framework of serving Christ's poor.

Pauper nurses (also known as 'wardsmaids' or 'wardsmen') were part of the nexus of institutionalised abjection and impotence that continued up to the final years of the workhouse in the 1920s. Lacking in skills, they made up for what they didn't know by utilising their 'lived experience' of the workhouse. But what most distinguished them from the other paupers was not their knowledge, character or virtues, but rather the fact that they had the physical strength to perform the tasks required of them (Twining, 1885, p 668). What exactly this meant can be gathered by an account of London's workhouse infirmaries, drawn up by Ernest Hart. In describing the nursing conducted by the pauper nurses in one infirmary, he wrote:

> The nurses generally had the most imperfect ideas of their duties.... One nurse plainly avowed that she gave medicines three times a day to those who were very ill, and twice or once a day as they improved. The medicines were given all down a ward in a cup; elsewhere in a gallipot. The nurse said she "poured out the medicine, and judged according." In other respects the nursing was equally deficient. The dressings were roughly and badly applied. Lotions and water dressings were applied in rags, which were allowed to dry and stick. I saw sloughing ulcers and cancers so treated. In fact, this was the rule. Bandages seemed to be unknown. But the general character of the nursing will be appreciated by the detail of one fact, that I found in one ward two paralytic patients with frightful sloughs of the back; they were both dirty, and lying on hard straw mattresses; the one dressed only with a rag steeped in chloride-of-lime solution, the other with a rag thickly covered with ointment. This latter was a fearful and very extensive sore, in a state of absolute putridity; the patient was covered with filth and excoriated, and the stench was masked by strewing dry chloride of lime on the floor under the bed. A spectacle more saddening or more discreditable cannot be imagined. Both these patients have since died. (Hart, 1866, pp 12-13)

Despite subsequent attempts to replace pauper nurses with trained or 'trainee' nurses, the new nurses were still seen as having 'low status, hard work, and unpleasant quarters' as well as minimal pay and training compared to those working in the voluntary hospitals (Crowther, 1982, p 187). When, in 1929, the Local Government Bill was passed, it ended the Poor Law unions and placed the institutions, their inmates and their staff under the responsibility of the local authority. The new public assistance committees that were set up in their place were accountable to the county councils and the borough councils (Longmate, 2003, p 278). Most of the plant and the labour – the institutions, the staff and the inmates – remained, however, and most people continued to think of them as the 'old' workhouse, up to and even beyond 1948 and the passing of National Assistance Act (Webster, 1991, pp 166-7).

As a result, long after the workhouses and their infirmaries were formally abolished, the buildings still provided 'the mainstay of local authority residential services for the handicapped and aged' (Townsend, 1962, p 63). There were few 'new builds'. The staff were not radically different from those of the old public assistance institutions. They consisted of a warden and/or matron, who were responsible for a few qualified nurses and a much larger number of attendants, cleaners, cooks and kitchen maids. Many 'residents' continued to provide services to their peers, much as the less infirm inmates had provided services to their more infirm peers during the previous 'Poor Law' era. Care work for frail older people remained institutionalised and subject to the same kind of scandal that had dogged the workhouse (Robb, 1967). Body work was either neglected or, if carried out, done so in a perfunctory and often inconsiderate manner (Townsend, 1962).

Changes were afoot. The Health Services and Public Health Act 1968 in England required local authorities to develop adequate community health and social services. While the implementation of the Act was delayed, by the mid to late 1970s there was a steady increase in the provision of home helps, home nurses, health visiting and various forms of day care that targeted older frail people (Bebbington, 1979). How far such work removed older people from the nexus of abjection associated with the institutions of the Poor Law was not always clear. A series of reports published from the 1970s onwards implied that institutional care remained unsatisfactory, and that 'community care' offered a much more satisfactory and less abject context for delivering intimate care (Meacher, 1972; Tobin and Lieberman, 1976; Clough, 1981; Booth, 1985). Research into the organisation, staffing and residents' degree of satisfaction with institutional nursing and residential care became a prominent feature of the 1980s, reflecting concerns over actual and potential abuse, and the limited qualifications and training of the domestic and care staff who were mostly responsible for looking after the residents and the home itself (Booth, 1985; Willcocks et al, 1987). But if the dominant focus of research into the care of the aged was on the 'quality' of care offered by the institution (or lack of it), the move toward a more explicitly consumerist model of care shifted the emphasis away from staff as a structural component of residential care (their morale, practices, qualifications, and training) to considering them as workers, focusing on the conditions and conflicts of their employment (Lee-Treweek, 1997).

Contemporary patterns of care work

As already noted, the nature of formal care work has suffered from the long shadows of the almshouse, the workhouse infirmary and all the other institutions designed to look after the aged and infirm. These were cast during the 19th and early 20th centuries, when the only formal alternative to institutional care was outdoor relief in the form of goods, money or other material benefits. During the first half of the 20th century such institutions played a relatively marginal role in the social relations of care. The extent and sheer size of the subsequent transformation of formal care work in the late 20th century is remarkable. In one study, conducted by Mignon Duffy and her colleagues in Massachusetts, USA, they found that, in the first decade of the 21st century, 20% of all adults' time was spent providing care to others. Nearly a quarter (22.4%) of the paid workforce in that state were employed in the care sector, and more than half (57%) of all state and local expenditure was directed toward providing or purchasing care activities (Duffy et al, 2013, p 161).

Duffy et al's study illustrates how care in its discrete and countable form consumes a greater amount of time and more resources than was ever the case in 'first modernity'. It plays a more important part than ever before, in shaping lives, fashioning identities and realising new social divides, and one can observe a take-off in research interest in this area over the course of the last two decades. This includes examination of the conflicted intimacies of 'body work' (Twigg, 2000), the demand for emotional labour as evidence of the 'quality of care' (James, 1992), and the continuing marginalisation of care workers themselves (Pollitt, 1990). A 2001 report from the Urban Institute in the US provides a particularly succinct outline of this latter point:

> Most paid providers of long-term care are paraprofessional workers. After informal caregivers, these workers are the most essential component in helping older persons and younger people with disabilities maintain some level of function and quality of life. According to recent US Bureau

of Labor Statistics (BLS) data, nursing assistants held about 750,000 jobs in nursing homes in 1998, while home health and personal care aides held about 746,000 jobs in that same year. Like informal caregivers, the overwhelming majority of frontline long-term care-workers are women. About 55 percent of nursing assistants are white, 35 percent are black, and 10 percent are Hispanic. Most workers are relatively disadvantaged economically and have low levels of educational attainment. While these paraprofessional workers are engaged in physically and emotionally demanding work, they are among the lowest paid in the service industry, making little more than the minimum wage. (Stone and Wiener, 2001, p 3)

In the UK, a recent examination of the long-term care workforce concluded that 'pay rates are among the lowest in the UK with the majority of wages on or near the National Minimum Wage' (Hussein et al, 2015, p 2). Not only are care workers paid near or below the minimum wage, but other aspects of their job also marginalise those who are already marginalised in other ways, with the result that turnover is high and shortages chronic (Hussein and Manthorpe, 2014). This renders the work even more demanding as existing staff struggle to cover absences and leave. Yet, despite the fact that the workforce is 'primarily female, middle-aged, ethnically diverse and poor' (Delp et al, 2010), and the demands and associated moral obligations are often burdensome (Aronson and Neysmith, 1997), studies examining 'job satisfaction' do not suggest a very dissatisfied or demoralised workforce (see, for example, Brodaty et al, 2003; Sims-Gould et al, 2010; Iecovich, 2011; Stone et al, 2013).

A constant theme in research into the work experience of people employed as aides, assistants, auxiliaries and/or domiciliary care workers is the attachments they form with the people they look after, and their consequent privileging of the intrinsic motivation for doing the job despite the weak extrinsic motivations of poor pay and conditions (Stone et al, 2013). This disparity (and the sense that women especially are prone to experiencing it) may provide further potential for the emotional and moral exploitation of the workforce (Himmelweit, 1999), but it also suggests that although 'body work' remains dirty work, performing it on other human bodies conveys a form of moral identity and sense of dignity from the exposure to such human vulnerability.

Unlike the care relationships that evolve between partners, parents and children, care work is from the start a more one-sided, functional relationship: someone gets paid to perform care; the work can be counted and its effects quantified; and whatever concerns there are can be framed in economic as much as in ethical terms (Himmelweit, 1999; Duffy et al, 2013). It is a major service industry – its organisation and management are accordingly big business (Folbre, 2012). In relation to home or institutional care directed toward infirm older people, the person being cared for is realised as a client because they are lacking the kind of pre-existing agency and identity that is attributed to others, including, of course, the care worker, his or her colleagues, employers and supervisors as well as other involved relatives, friends and neighbours. The carer's identity as carer is that of a worker, paid very often as an unskilled, manual labourer, but nevertheless imbued with qualities that are also considered 'caring' (Rainbird et al, 1999). The methods, motivations, practices and 'quality standards' of care workers are subject to more analysis than that of 'informal' carers whose care is seen as a function of his or her shared history with the person being cared for and their affective, social and physical proximity.

The experience of care and care work

While research into the informal care of frail older people has concentrated heavily on the burden and stresses of such care faced by carers and the factors ameliorating or exacerbating that burden (Pinquart and Sörensen, 2003; Sörensen and Conwell, 2011), formal care work has not been analysed in such terms. Instead, the focus has more often been on the tasks of care, how well they are performed and the terms and conditions of the workers (Lee-Treweek, 1997; Stacey, 2011; Palmer and Eveline, 2012). There is a noticeable absence of any analysis of what it is like caring or being cared for in formal care settings. Even in the limited research that has been conducted on the experience of care work, emphasis has been on the agency and subjectivity of the care workers, their experiences, the rewarding and stressful aspects of their job, and the 'caring ethic' they should or do employ. The person being cared for is, by and large, no more considered as co-constructor of the care relationship than is a house or a carpet needing to be cleaned and dusted, yet this is what is most feared by older people contemplating their future self in care (Harrefors et al, 2009).

The cared for older person is *not* not considered, of course, but such consideration that is given is framed not in agentic terms, but rather in terms of older people as potential subjects of suffering. Thus residents (or their proxies) are interrogated as to whether the quality of their life has been improved, whether their health or functioning is being maintained, whether they have been prevented from falling and whether or not their 'personhood' has been maintained and their 'dignity' enhanced (Hall and Høy, 2012). Care workers, by contrast, are not examined along similar parameters – they are not viewed as suffering subjects, and certainly not viewed as having experienced any enhancement of their dignity or personhood as a result of their care work. Instead, their labour is measured in terms of the tasks performed and the manner in which they perform them. The differential placing of agency, identity and subjectivity reflect the power imbalances between the positions of carers and those being cared for, and the different moral identities assigned to worker and to resident. The result is that those aspects of care that both share, in terms of living and working under the shadows of abjection and the adversities of care and the daily struggle to find meaning in the care of strangers, are strangely ignored.

This two-dimensional portrait of care work can be contrasted with that of work concerning 'people with disabilities', a group that, while formally including older people receiving formal care, manages, nevertheless, to exclude them. 'People with disabilities' can be seen as an identity increasingly imbued with agency and autonomy, an identity constructed with not wanting care or compassion, but out of the demand for a fair deal. At the centre of disability studies is the assumption that people with disabilities need to be approached and studied as agents, with their desires and wants as well as their experiences of exclusion and oppression being subject to examination and exploration. As Bill Hughes and his colleagues have noted, people in the disability movement have tended to steer clear of the topic of care (Hughes et al, 2005), arguably because they believe that the discourse of care tends either to advance the perspective of professionals and providers or to valorise the virtues of giving care, leaving the care recipient less agentic, less valued and more marginal (Hughes et al, 2005).

Given the caution surrounding any interrogation of care work that risks representing people with disabilities as the objects of care, such research that has been conducted pursues a different agenda, focusing instead on the experience of being cared for, the subjectivity of being looked on and looked after, as well as the burdensomeness of being aware that one is being cared for (Galvin, 2004; Charmaz, 2008). In addition, the disability movement has emphasised the 'power of personal experience' and the expertise that this confers (Morris, 2001, p 5), consequently making it much harder for research to explore the experience of formal and informal care without reference to the subjectivities of the people being cared for. While it can be argued that such a perspective has tended to emphasise access, control and rights over subjectivity and experience, what it has also achieved is to constrain those research agendas that construct care from an exclusive preoccupation with objective indicators of need, the subjective experience of carers or the social organisation of care work, insisting on 'caring as a site of subjectivity' (Chattoo and Ahmad, 2008, p 551).

Research into the care of frail older people has experienced less constraint; given the dominant position of people with dementia in this literature, it is understandable that the voice of the frail older person being cared for has rarely been sought. Influenced by the disability studies tradition, attempts to change the focus and introduce the voice of 'the user' or 'client' have begun, not just in care work, but more generally in all areas of human services research (Hubbard et al, 2003). Despite the good intentions of such researchers, however, the methods of 'including' the person with dementia tend to be determined by the ingenuity and interpretive skills of the researchers and their interviewers rather than the urgency of older people with dementia to voice their concerns and desires for care or their irritations with it. Although there are some attempts to promote peer advocacy movements in this area (Bryden, 2015), and even more tentative initiatives to involve people with dementia as peer researchers, this work is still at a very early stage (Tanner, 2012). The appearance of autobiographical accounts of people with the diagnosis of Alzheimer's might seem to provide an alternative arena for exploring the subjectivity of care, but most such accounts have been given by middle-aged people whose need for support for 'self-care' at the time of writing was quite minimal (Page and Keady, 2010). Consequently, their main focus has been on coming to terms with the diagnosis, preservation of autonomy and identity as well as their own coping with the consequent impairments.

Care work and care homes

Given these caveats, it is important to distinguish research that has focused on the differing experiences of people who have been 'placed' in care and living in care homes, and people who anticipate becoming sufficiently dependent to have to 'go' into care and who may well fear the abjection that a nursing home seems to realise, as well as those elderly people who choose to enter residential care as a way of not burdening their family or of increasing their sense of security and reducing their sense of social isolation. While the threshold for publicly funding residential care has increasingly restricted paying for such accommodation to the more abjectly frail, it is still the case that some private residential homes, and even some nursing homes, continue to provide places for some older people who have not yet become so frail as to be unable to articulate their desire for the company of others or the security of being in a 'home'. In such cases, there remains the possibility of experiencing more company than care (Rodriguez-Martin et al, 2014).

Nevertheless, it is care rather than company that dominates the rationale of the nursing home, and it is unsurprising that the desire for, and the experience of, being 'in a home' is generally less central to the aims, virtues and moral necessity of care home work and to those who research it. Despite recognising that care is a form of social relationship, ethicists and professionals alike have treated institutional care as a set of practices or regimes that are dominated by the agency and identity of the carers — and indirectly, of those who manage the carers. Even if its virtue is determined by the extent to which it is directed toward the agency and autonomy of the person being cared for, such an ethos presented by the home and its representatives still treats the potential resident as at most a passive consumer of 'person-centred' or 'dignified' care, the nature of which is underwritten by the manager or senior staff of the institution. The inevitable asymmetry in the relationship is amplified by institutional-based care work, and is less easily recognised resisted or reflected on by those whose social identity is embodied within such regimes.

Studies of nursing home residents who are neither seriously impaired nor deemed to suffer from dementia provide some insight into the subjective experience of the care home regime. What such studies suggest is that the care relationship — that is, the relations with care staff — provides the most notable focus for people's experiences, both bad and good, of the nursing home (Grau et al, 1997). Another study also found that most residents interviewed saw care largely through the medium of their relationships with staff, but the authors observed significant minorities who saw it either as a 'service' or as providing (or failing to provide) comfort, safety and security (Bowers et al, 2001). Unsurprisingly the view of 'care-as-service' was expressed by people who were largely funding their own care, while the 'care-as-comfort' was a view expressed by more disabled and dependent residents. Other studies reinforce the view that for residents it is their relationship with care staff that plays a critical role in reducing their sense of abjection, vulnerability and helplessness that otherwise surrounds them in the nursing home (Nakrem et al, 2011, 2013). While funding one's own nursing home care might offer some people the opportunity to retain a degree of control and power within their relationship with staff, for the majority of residents their sense of self and security rests heavily on what one writer has called the 'organized emotional care' that is provided by the staff themselves (Lopez, 2006). The extent to which the fiscal and resource constraints of the nursing home industry gives workers the freedom and organisational support to express what Lopez terms 'emotional authenticity' is obviously important, but the importance for both residents and workers to be free to express their feelings and to realise their respective moral identities can scarcely be disputed.

Care work and the transformation of home

If the nursing home has come to symbolise the alienation and otherness of deep old age within its particular set of social relations of care, how might we understand the social relations of formal care provided to older persons in their own home? The denser and darker the picture drawn of nursing home care, the more desirable it seems for people in later life to stay 'at home', no matter what. The long shadow of impoverishment and shame associated with being brought to the almshouse or workhouse has not disappeared; arguably, it has been augmented or replaced by the shame associated with a lack of both corporeal integrity and social integration. Frailty is now one of the major social divisions in later life, contrasting the success of being a fully paid up member of the third age with the shamefacedness of a failed body, a failing mind and failing family support (Gilleard and Higgs, 2016). Under such circumstances, managing to stay at home might seem to offer some kind of bulwark against going into a home. The vulnerability of growing mental and physical infirmity, however, threatens in a more insidious way any sense of 'at homeness' that a fit body, agile mind and social connectedness more powerfully confers.

The concept of 'at homeness' has been recently reviewed in a series of Swedish studies examining 'at homeness despite illness and disease' (Őhlén et al, 2014). These authors considered three aspects of being symbolically at home – the feeling of being safe, of being connected and of being centred (Őhlén et al, 2014, p 6). How far home-based care facilitates such sentiments and how far it may further undermine them is a question that cannot be easily answered, but arguably it provides a focus through which home care can be explored. While the social relations of 'informal' care emerge out of other identities and other relationships in which the older person might reasonably be expected to be at home, and where the stresses and strains of caring join together as much as they separate carer and cared for, home-based formal care work is 'essentialised' as reproductive labour, abstracted from any complications of past relations, past identities or indeed, of past connections. To that extent it is alien, an intrusion into the life-world of people who are feeling increasingly unsafe – losing trust in both their bodies and their minds.

While there are no doubt important structural differences between the various sectors involved in the domiciliary care industry, our main focus is on the generic features of such care and its contribution to maintaining the sense of at homeness and offsetting the vulnerability of frailty to the shadow of the fourth age's social imaginary. Aside from the social policy issues of funding and organising these sectors of domiciliary care, three themes seem apparent in the research literature on home care: namely, the motivations and moral identities of care workers; the tasks, challenges and stresses home care workers face; and the care relationship itself, whether contrasted explicitly with informal, family care, or explored directly.

Care work, care ethos and the moral order of care

It is generally accepted that the frail aged person being cared for is no more equivalent to a rubbish tip being scoured for its plastic or metal content than he or she is the equivalent of a baby. Care work is not 'dirty work' devoid of human meaning (Anderson, 2000), but neither is it the intrinsically 'nurturing' labour that is witness to human growth and flourishing. Representing long-term care as a nexus of pure abjection needs to be qualified just as does representing it as a labour of love and compassion. It is unlikely that all pauper nurses, or wardsmen and women of the Victorian infirmary, were pitiless, uncaring *lumpen*. It is equally unlikely that the attachments that arise in care work can ever be replicas of other familial relationships. In the conflicting arena between intimacy and abjection, closeness and incapacity, the identity and otherness of the person being cared for seems to form an uncertain dialectic with the moral identity of the care worker, the outcome of which may strongly determine how much damage caring does and how much protection it affords.

Care work varies along a number of parameters, one of which seems very different from other forms of domestic service – that is the intrinsic motivation that is assumed among those choosing to perform care work. While cleaners, gardeners, hairdressers and personal trainers may all want to do and be seen to do a good job, what constitutes a good job is usually determined by some end-product such as a clean floor, a neatly mown garden, a stylish haircut or a fitter client. There is generally little expectation that the service provider should be anything more than courteous and efficient in performing their task. With care, however, there are other expectations that arise because the person being cared for rather than just being serviced is someone in need, someone potentially suffering, someone who does not have the everyday capabilities of a working person, parent or senior citizen. Their identity is shaped by this moral dimension of care and its echoes with 'family'.

While the abject work of domestic servants or those whose livelihoods require them daily to dig deep into what society has discarded can be said to constitute forms of 'dirty work', the essential humanity – personhood – of frail older people makes it much harder to treat care work simply as undignified dirty work. The expectation in providing care is that one is helping somebody and helping is inherently deemed virtuous. Care work is generally regarded as a worthy, if not well paid, job, one that it is performed as much out of care and concern as for the money (England et al, 2012). While many of those engaged in care work are not regarded as 'professionals', many others are. Nurses, social workers, therapists and healthcare (or nursing) assistants each have varying degrees of professional qualification, compared with home or personal care workers or home care aides. As a consequence, in addition to (and perhaps in place of) the moral imperative of care, professionalised care workers can draw on and be socialised into a set of values that their professional organisations articulate in training, regularly reinforce in post-qualification reviews and become the subject of peer discussions and formal supervision, as well as being a factor in negotiations over pay and conditions.

At the same time, long-term care overlaps with other forms of domestic work that are more exploitative and damaging (Anderson, 2000). One area of overlap, for example, is the physical and verbal abuse that both domestic and long-term care workers not infrequently report from the person receiving their services (Somboontanont et al, 2007; Isaksson et al, 2009; Lachs et al, 2013). Although not a topic easy to research – not least because of the implications such reporting may have for staff – the complex inter-dependency between the abuse experienced and the abuse practised by residents and staff, carers and cared for, is now beginning to be explored (Malmedal et al, 2014). Abuse and intimate relationships are often closely related, and the existence of affection and inter-dependency in the carer/cared for nexus is no protection from either abjection or abuse. In our earlier chapter on abjection (see Chapter 5), we noted how the care nexus retains a dual identity – as both a site of moral desert as well as one of disgust. Rodriquez (2011) has noted the way nursing home care workers articulated a moral order in that nexus by selectively advancing those aspects of agency and identity that gave value to the residents while denying agency to those destructive or undignified acts that threatened the moral identity of both resident and care worker.

While the professionalisation of nurses, therapists and others working in nursing homes can serve as one means of maintaining a valued identity in the job of caring, those care workers lacking access to such narratives must draw on other non-professionalised discourses. These range from the selective attributions of agency to residents that was noted by Rodriquez, to the use of 'family' metaphors to describe their care and those they care for (Berdes and Eckert, 2007; Dodson and Zincavage, 2007). Such narratives seem to arise regularly within the nursing home setting, and arguably act both as a common template for caring in general and as a deterrent against staff abuse, neglect and 'objectification' (Ashforth and Kreiner, 1999). However, unlike the selective positioning of identity associated with professionalised discourse, such common templates as the 'family' metaphor may inadvertently promote moral identity conflicts with the residents' actual families. This can create a sort of competition between 'real' and 'imagined' family over who now 'knows' the resident best (Abrahamson et al, 2007). Visiting family members may be judged by care staff to no longer share the same relationship with the person who is now a resident that they once did, leading family members in turn to feel they are losing any position of primacy as 'carer', and to search instead for faults that threaten or undermine the care workers' status.

How far a more professionalised discourse prevents a descent into abjection, abuse or both, and how far it can reduce the conflicts of care are perhaps unanswerable questions. Framing caring as central to the professional ethos of nursing or emphasising 'person-centred' care in professionalised dementia care seems to imply that such an ethos can carry with it the obvious benefit of improved care. By eliding aspects of what might be termed 'affective' labour, with instrumental 'competence' and specialist 'knowledge', the professional care worker (and her or his team) is expected to deliver better care, which, it is presumed, will benefit the wellbeing of the residents. The benchmark is not high. One early observational study, using standardised measures of 'dementia care', found that neither public nor private care homes provided 'even a fair standard of care' (Ballard et al, 2001, p 426). Using a randomised control methodology, an attempt was made to compare the effectiveness of person-centred care, dementia care mapping (a more structured form of person-centred care) and care as usual in 15 care homes in Australia. Although both the 'person-centred' regimes seemed to have reduced levels of agitation compared with 'care as usual', there was no evidence that these specialist practices had any other effects, either on measures of quality of life, observed neuropsychiatric symptomatology, drug use or falls (Chenoweth et al, 2009). A subsequent review of this area pointed out the complexity of what is meant by person-centred care, and how it is realised, with the result that it has proved difficult to evaluate (Brownie and Nancarrow, 2013).

While some have argued that introducing 'culture change' into nursing homes brings benefits to staff as well as residents, it could also be argued that those with the least power and status (that is, the least professionalised) benefit least from such innovations, and may possibly find the change unsettling rather than empowering (Palmer et al, 2013). Whether culture change within nursing homes improves the subjective experiences of residents is difficult to ascertain; whether it benefits staff is a more realisable task. If, at the very least, the instrumental competence of care workers can be improved (whether to dress wounds, minimise use of psychotropic drugs, prevent ulcers and falls, or reduce tube feeding and the use of restraints), without compromising the moral framework of care, it is clearly worth making the effort, even if the effects can be assessed only by care workers perceiving themselves as better (Miller et al, 2013).

Conclusions

Care work has become a major service industry, the terms and conditions of which have an impact beyond the workforce to touch an ever larger number of families. Caught between the life-world of the family and the system world of managed labour, so to speak, the identity of care workers is split between the moral imperatives of care located within the household and the contractual and professional frameworks of wage labour. This, in turn, reflects on the identity of those who are the objects of care, increasingly those infirm older people whose lack of capital – whether viewed in its cultural, financial or social forms – places them in the position of having their personhood identified and attributed by the practices of the care workers and the narratives of those who manage that care. The kind of body work that is performed, as well as the abjection surrounding it, makes the job difficult. Historically, such formal care work has lacked status, echoing the tasks once performed by unpaid, untrained pauper nurses in the workhouse infirmaries.

Yet care work also contains a moral identity, reflecting other practices and other relationships, of the reciprocal relationships of care and support expected of family and kin. That formal care frequently first supplements then takes over from informal care only reinforces the similarity, while introducing a distinction based not just, or not even, on pay, but on the 'otherness' that is introduced into the care relationship as carer and cared for meet each other as strangers. That strangeness is perhaps already prefigured in the gradual estrangement that takes place during the evolution of informal care relationships, as the reciprocity between partners or between parents and children is gradually recalibrated toward a relationship of one. But just as it is possible to witness affection, moral identity and social reciprocity within informal care relationships, so, too, do the formal relationships of long-term care retain the possibility of realising those features, even though it may be harder. This is especially true if the person being cared for has increasing difficulties in reflecting on themselves, their limitations as well as the performances required of them – in order to aid, appreciate and acknowledge their role as an understanding care recipient. As infirmity increases and the resources to continue to 'co-construct' the care relationship diminishes, formal care takes on wider responsibilities to shape what goes on, to what ends and through which forms of agency.

Research on long-term care has proved difficult to conduct and to provide an empirical demonstration of what constitutes 'good' care. Perhaps such consequentialist strategies can never provide a satisfactory answer because the question is one of moral identity rather than social effectiveness. As the economic values of the market or of a residualised welfare policy come to shape the debate over long-term care, research will no doubt continue to seek out appropriate answers. But in the everyday practices of care, resort will still be made to the life-world values of the family, of obligation and reciprocity. Good care, in these terms, is care provided by people who are driven by a moral imperative – not just to do, but to be good. In a world where universalist claims are viewed as suspect, considering what it means to do a good job and to be a good carer requires the space and opportunity to reflect on the job, to feel that others respect you for respecting such values, and to acknowledge that good intentions are themselves never enough.

EIGHT

Care without limits

In the previous two chapters we addressed the nature of care, conceptualised variously as a labour of love, a contractual relationship, a professional practice or as a moral and material imperative. While we have represented the person being cared for as already old, frail and potentially abject, we have recognised that the degree of any person's 'frailure' can be magnified or minimised by the narratives and practices of care within which their frailty is embedded. While pervasively present within any care relationship, the social imaginary of the fourth age can be challenged, kept at bay or actively resisted, just as it can be brought down further and made even darker. Care cannot eliminate this imaginary; it is of necessity oriented towards it. This is so both in the transitions of pre-existing family relationships into the more focused relationships of 'informal care' as it is in the targeted insertion of 'formal care' into the everyday lives of frailed older people. Although such transformations remain sources of troubled subjectivities, they are not without scope for negotiation. In such contexts of change and transition, there is always some prospect of mitigation, some element, however slight, of finding or maintaining a redeeming and reciprocal relationship. In this chapter we turn to issues of providing care 'at the limits' of any possible social relationship – care provided to those whose lives seem surrounded on all sides by the more impenetrable aspects of the fourth age's social imaginary.

In describing the care of people in such situations it is important not to lose sight of the distinction between a shared social imaginary of the fourth age and the corporeal realities that are experienced by individual frail older people and their difficult and disadvantaged lives. However, we would contend that it is impossible to escape the power of the various discourses that surround these individuals, even if these discourses can never fully represent the everyday practices of care or the experiences of bodily distress. The practices of care can never be reduced to a single discourse any more than care can be reduced to a single ethic or virtue. At most it is only possible to pursue an open dialogue between these two phenomena – between the corporeality of caring and the discourses and practices of care oriented toward that corporeality.

Writing about care at its limits, it is first of all important to define what limits we are referring to. By care at its limits we mean care that is performed for persons whose social, psychic and human qualities are deemed by others (usually, but not necessarily, including the care worker[s] themselves) to be utterly dependent on the provision of care. While this will inevitably conjure up in each reader a slightly different example, our intended focus is on those older people exhibiting the most profound degree of mental and physical infirmity; people with advanced or severe dementia; those seriously disabled by stroke; or individuals who are otherwise incapacitated by end stage disease. Up until this point we have written of care being realised within the shadows of the fourth age imaginary. We have not written of care taking place *within* the fourth age. While the discourses and practices of care in later life are influenced by the infirmities of the person being cared for, they are never fully determined by them. Numerous regional and international studies of variations in care demonstrate this point, as does even a cursory examination of changing practices over time. There will always appear to be possibilities of care that keep the care recipient at a distance from such shadowy imaginations. Unbuttoning unobtrusively a difficult button, making sure a bottom is carefully cleaned, waiting patiently for a mouthful of food to be swallowed – in these and many other ways carers can and do 'credit' the person they are looking after with concerns, desires, fears and sensitivities of equivalent significance as their own. However ephemeral to the plans, practices and performances of the carer and the moral status of the care recipient's personhood, 'doing care right' can seem to make the fourth age imaginary only an option, something avoidable, allowing carers to 'co-construct' care for both themselves and the people they care for.

But are such possibilities always possible? What about those circumstances when attributions of agency seem completely implausible, when the care encounter is realised almost entirely by the acts and narratives of the carer and those who share in or witness their care, as when, for example, a nursing home resident is maintained under deep sedation until death? Is there no limit to the social relations or co-construction of care? Not even when the person being cared for seems to have disappeared into the 'black hole' of the fourth age, when both their agency and their identity can only be imagined? These are the issues we explore in the following pages. To begin with, we consider the journeys through which some older people reach ever more advanced or severe stages of mental and bodily infirmity.

Journeys towards advanced infirmity

More than any other chronic illness or condition, dementia affects older people's capacity to perform the activities of daily life, and it is the loss of these skills that are most likely to lead to care in a long-term care facility or institution (Aguero-Torres et al, 2001; Bharucha et al, 2004; von Bonsdorff et al, 2006; Puts et al, 2005; Luppa et al, 2008). Across Europe and North America, in Australia and in many industrialised East Asian countries, the majority of people with advanced dementia will spend their last few months or years not at home, but in a nursing home or hospital, where they will be cared for by strangers (Smith et al, 2000; Mitchell et al, 2005; Houttekier et al, 2010). Although this 'transition' does not usually constitute an end of 'informal' caring, it does alter the nature of care and the social identities of both carers and care recipients.

Severe decline in mental and physical functioning makes it hard (if not impossible) for informal carers – partners, adult children or other friends of family – to maintain either the household of the infirm older person, or, if sharing that household, the 'at homeness' of the infirm older person him- or herself. Most of the older people admitted with a diagnosis of dementia into a nursing home or similar long-stay care facility are not abandoned by their friends and family. The transition is rarely so abrupt or final, and many informal carers find it very hard to 'let go' of their partner or parent, continuing to visit even when they are no longer recognised or acknowledged by their relative (Hennings et al, 2013). Still, the move into 'care' represents a major transition, a further stage in a journey that leads from a shared identity located in familiar relationships towards a barer and bleaker relationship fashioned within the nursing home or equivalent long-term care facility (Førsund et al, 2015).

Not everyone who develops dementia ends up in long-term care, and not everyone who ends up in long-term care is suffering from dementia. Other conditions can lead to similar outcomes. To what extent should we assume that the course of advanced dementia represents a template for all forms of 'end stage' care? In our earlier chapter on 'frailty' (see Chapter 4), we addressed the literature on chronic illness and multi-morbidity in later life. We did so largely from an epidemiological perspective, noting how with increasing age morbidity increases and multiplies. With age, the course of chronic disease blurs within the intersecting discourses of multiple diseases and multidimensional impairments. There is an assumption – not so far disproven – that a common progression of disabilities occurs in the frailing of old age, beginning with difficulties in performing the instrumental activities of daily life, such as managing household accounts, cleaning or shopping, moving on to the failure to adequately perform such basic self-care activities as bathing, dressing, washing or the use of the toilet, and ending with utter dependency.

This narrative based on the use of measures of instrumental and self-care activities of daily life frames the person with infirmity as an increasingly dependent person needing an increasing amount of care. It relies on assessing or staging incapacity by degrees, and is typically based on others' observations. A less objectifying way of representing the course of chronic illness has been framed through the concept of a 'disrupted biographical narrative' (Bury, 1982; Williams, 1984, 2000). At first this research assumed a 'normal' life course, whose biography is first disrupted and then reconstructed, taking account and making sense of the experience of change that arises when one experiences chronic illness as well as impairment (Bury, 1982). Subsequent accounts have questioned the unitary nature of such narratives, especially when set in the context of ageing and later life where multiple narratives are represented (Cornwell, 1984). Although some conditions like stroke seem to conform to the 'disrupted' biography model (Salter et al, 2008), others seem more aligned to narratives that represent the condition as an assault, the victim of which is deemed a sort of foot soldier in the battle against the condition. This is exemplified in many subjective accounts of cancer (Mathieson and Stam, 1995; Hubbard and Forbat, 2012). Other researchers have observed that many progressive but relatively unobtrusive conditions, such as chronic obstructive pulmonary disease (COPD), end stage kidney disease or type II diabetes are framed as just one of the less fortunate ways that some people grow older (Pinnock et al, 2011; Llewellyn et al, 2014; Low et al, 2014). Growing older, uncomfortably, may seem the more apt narrative for the person affected and for their family since it helps naturalise their condition, and constitutes a kind of continuity in the identity of the relationship as one of caring for *my* partner/parent in *her* or *his* old age (Elofsson and Öhlén, 2004).

Transfer to formal care poses a severe threat to such narrative continuities. It can be imagined that losing one's home and confronting the reduced autonomy, limited possibilities for negotiation and constant exposure of one's vulnerabilities to younger, fitter others is harder for individuals to accommodate. There is limited research into the experiences of older infirm people being cared for in advanced stages of ill health moving into and renegotiating their identity in the long-term care setting. What research there is pinpoints the importance given to retaining the ability – and the opportunity – for such care recipients to express aspects of their identity, to exercise in however limited a way some degree of agency, as well as to experience in one form or another some sense of being cared for and cared about – and ideally from people for whom one also cares about (Andersson et al, 2007). While it may be glib to insist that such opportunities can always be realised, especially in end stage disease, it remains the case that when asked, infirm older people do still articulate such views. Studies show that people with 'sound minds' give importance to maintaining a sense of dignity in the face of ever increasing dependency, and arguably the same might be assumed for people in long-term care who suffer from severe dementia; they, too, want to be cared for, while at the same time being 'treated as adult and accountable persons' (von Kutzleben et al, 2012, p 385). The potential conflict between these two sets of needs, of being cared for and of being treated as an adult, is evident. The capacity of people with severe or advanced dementia to negotiate between these competing interests is much weaker compared with older people with other severe or advanced chronic conditions. Yet ironically, such negotiations are probably more necessary, given the greater difficulties that people with advanced dementia have in asserting and sustaining agency and identity (Clare, 2010). The position of such individuals might seem to be that said by Baltes to characterise the fourth age, namely, possessing an increased dependency on culture and society concomitant with a reduced capacity to benefit from these external sources (Baltes and Smith, 2003).

Similar themes of wanting to be cared for without sacrificing a sense of agency and autonomy have been reported in other studies (Hall et al, 2009; Anderberg and Berglund, 2010). In a study of Swedish nursing home residents, one of the residents commented to the researchers:

> Do you know what makes me happy? To be able to go to the toilet on my own. It gives me satisfaction not having to ask for help with everything. I'm so grateful that I can take care of myself as much as I can. (quoted in Dwyer et al, 2008, p 101)

Given the difficulties in meeting these kinds of concerns and interests in cases of advanced dementia, how possible and practical is it to not just assume an equivalence of such interests but to realise them in care?

Mapping versus storying 'decline'

Before exploring in more detail the possibilities and constraints in providing care to people with advanced or end stage dementia, while realising agency and autonomy, again, we must try to be as clear as we can about our terminology. This takes us back to the task of 'staging dementia'. Given the limited possibilities for exploring the journey into advanced dementia as a 'disrupted biographical narrative', there are two other possible routes. One seeks to account for the journey by tracking its pathological course as a staged decline into severe dependency (McLaughlin et al, 2010), while the other seeks to reconstruct the process not as autobiography, but as a kind of biography, drawing on some combination of early subjective accounts, supplemented at later stages by proxy accounts drawn from friends, relatives and carers of people with dementia (Harris, 2002; de Boer et al, 2007). Given the weight of research that has taken the former approach, we begin with objective accounts of staging dementia.

Most of the initial attempts to describe the symptomatic and pathological markers of the progress of dementia were undertaken before contemporary clinical treatment-oriented research began in the late 1970s and early 1980s. They were characterised by attempts to demonstrate significant co-variation between post-mortem confirmed brain pathology and the degree of cognitive impairment observed in life, relying on scores on mental status tests assessing cognitive function (Blessed et al, 1968). Following the development of the cholinergic hypothesis of dementia in the late 1970s (Perry, 1986), the pharmaceutical industry developed numerous potential candidate drugs for anti-dementia therapy. These were designed along the lines established for the treatment of Parkinson's disease as a specific dopaminergic deficiency disease (Whitehouse, 1993). As a consequence of these developments, studies began to fashion clinical methods of 'staging' dementia in order to assess the relative effectiveness of the new 'anti-dementia' drugs in delaying or preventing further deterioration.

Among the best known of these were the Clinical Dementia Rating Scale (CDR) (Hughes et al, 1982) and the Global Deterioration Scale (GDS) (Reisberg et al, 1982). Both measures defined several stages of dementia: the CDR employs a number of criteria to define each stage such as cognition, personal care, home activities and interests, and social engagement. It ranged from a score of 0.5 indicating 'questionable' dementia, through to mild (CDR 1.0), moderate (CDR 2.0) and severe (CDR 3.0). By comparison, the GDS relied primarily on tests of mental functioning and had seven stages. Three of these were framed as precursor stages: from normal (DRS 1) to age-related memory problems (DRS 2) to borderline dementia (DRS 3), while the other four more or less follow the same grading system as the CDR. Criticisms of these scales began to emerge when longitudinal studies suggested that not all 'questionable' degrees of impairment transitioned into dementia, and not all forms of cognitive and behavioural decline in mild to moderate dementia, followed a simple model of linear decrement (Eisdorfer et al, 1992; Rabheru, 2007). Only later did interest extend beyond the stages of dementia that were of primary pharmacotherapeutic interest, as researchers began to consider later transition from moderate to severe dementia and the final pathway of severe or advanced dementia. In 2009, Mitchell and her colleagues complained that despite all the research into dementia, it was still the case that 'the clinical course of advanced dementia has not been described in a rigorous prospective manner' (Mitchell et al, 2009, p 1530). They employed Reisberg's DRS scale to select nursing home residents rates as 'severe' (DRS 7), and followed these people for 18 months, during which time over half died and many experienced increasingly unpleasant physical symptoms such as breathlessness, pain, pressure ulcers, aspiration and agitation during what was deemed this 'terminal' phase.

Aside from the early recognition that patterns of change can be very unpredictable and that not all aspects of cognition and self-care decline at a similar, constant rate, it also became clear that other so-called psychopathological features associated with dementia showed an even more variable pattern, appearing and disappearing throughout the course of dementia (Hope et al, 1997; Eustace et al, 2002; Aalten et al, 2005). Whether either psychopathology or physical pathology are necessary accompaniments to the underlying dementia was difficult to establish. Problems seemed to emerge at different times and with different implications, some making care for the person harder (usually psychopathology), while others (usually physical pathology) made care, if not more straightforward, at least more understandable to the carers.

Studies of the progress of dependency and the accumulation of symptoms of ill health such as aspiration, dyspnoea, eating difficulties, pain and sleeplessness seem to provide a common pathway, linking the progress of dementia with the generic decline associated with 'frailty as a long term condition' (Harrison et al, 2015). However, there seem to be clear differences both in the rate and the degree of dependency during the last two years of life. While infirm older people without dementia show a faster rate but lesser degree of dependency, people with dementia show a slower rate but greater degree (Covinsky et al, 2003; Chen et al, 2007). By implication, people with chronic infirmities without mental infirmity remain more independent and more able to do things for themselves than people with dementia. Consequently they seem to have more capacity to demonstrate their agency and to assert their identity despite living in long-term care. The course of end stage dementia is more profoundly disabling and exhibits fewer options to express identity or demonstrate agency, and by implication for people with dementia to be able to resist the pull of the fourth age. These objective accounts of end stage dementia suggest that it is a more profoundly difficult and helpless condition than that associated with other chronic disabling disorders. Whether it is also more distressing an experience for the person is open to greater doubt. While it is clear that it may be, for example, based on the distress reported by people in the earlier stages of dementia, when narrative accounts are more easily expressed and rendered understandable (Jetten et al, 2010), the distress may become less if, at later stages, the desire to be someone fades.

In contrast to the large body of research mapping the stages and progression of dementia and other sources of late life infirmity, narrative accounts of that journey are uncommon. In one study of residents with dementia living in care homes, Surr observed that '… [d]espite having memory problems many of the participants still appeared to be generating a life story and to be setting their present experiences in the context of their past in order to maintain a sense of self' (Surr, 2006, p 1728). The transcripts reported in that study suggest a somewhat fragile grasp of their circumstances. Mostly they focused on accounts of past or present relationships rather than on the journey that had brought the residents into the home. Clearly there were many in the homes unable to provide any coherent account or story. Reviews of the capacity of people with severe or moderate to severe dementia to represent themselves, narrate their journey or reflect on their circumstances suggest that people with severe dementia have at least a moderately disturbed, and many a severely disturbed, awareness of their cognitive disabilities, despite normal levels of conscious awareness (Clare, 2010, p 29). While it is possible to glean evidence of first-person accounts from persons with severe dementia, such accounts represent more a past self – Ricoeur's *idem* – rather than the changing biography of the present self – Ricoeur's *ipse* (Ricoeur, 1992).

The capacity to narrate the journey into dementia seems to be limited to journeys made during the earlier stages of dementia, and it may not be possible to generalise from such accounts of the progress into dementia to the experience of progressing to severe or end stage dementia (Page and Keady, 2010). Arguably it is at the advanced stages of dementia that one can consider the person coming closest to the event horizon, that edge of the metaphorical black hole of the fourth age (Gilleard and Higgs, 2010). From here little light is reflected; what emerges are the speculations, hopes and attributions of others. Whether these are family, friends, carers or researchers, inevitably these are third-person accounts. The model of the disrupted biographical narrative seems no longer to hold; it might better be replaced by the image of an orphaned body whose future must be held and told by others to others (Higgs and Gilleard, 2014).

Advanced dementia, terminal personhood

Most people with advanced dementia are unable to sustain a narrative of their circumstances, nor are they able to represent with any consistency to either themselves or others their experiences, nor are such persons able to negotiate a dialogue that could place them between a self, with recognised autonomy and an other that feels safely cared for. We – the carers, clinicians, family, fellow residents, students and researchers – are at best looking through a mirror darkly, relying on our own and others narratives that we believe share roughly the same sense of the direction of travel (Schubert et al, 2006). For many family members, such a view can be one drenched with unhappiness (Hennings et al, 2013). But for care workers, narratives attributing agency, intent and identity persist. In his account of a participant observation study in two nursing homes in the US, Jason Rodriquez outlined the ways care workers assert agency 'unto death' among nursing home residents, at the same time denying any such agency or intent to the uglier struggles that arise over care (Rodriquez, 2014, pp 139-54). Agency, he argues, is deployed as a rhetorical resource, attributed or denied to residents in a way that sustains their and their care worker's moral identities (Rodriquez, 2014, pp 151-4).

In much of the writing on 'dementia care', a central concern has been on asserting and enhancing the agency, identity and integrity of the person with dementia while trying to ensure they feel safe secure and as free as possible from unnecessary suffering (Adams, 2008; Lawrence et al, 2012). In the light of research noted above, this might seem a reasonable strategy to employ. Less attention has been paid to what might be called the 'terminal care' of dementia where agency and identity are harder to demonstrate let alone enhance, and suffering may seem difficult to detect or relieve. Such studies are beginning to appear, and it is to their consideration that we next turn, in considering the limits of care at the limits of personhood. Before we do so, it is important to acknowledge that many still dispute whether dementia should be treated as a terminal condition, claiming that 'patients die with the disease, not directly of it' (McCarthy et al, 1997, p 404; Goodman et al, 2010, p 330). For whatever reason, 'little research has focused on the detail of the experiences of patients with dementia and their carers leading up to the last days of life' (Goodman et al, 2010, p 335). Whether it is terminal in more than a descriptive sense may not be answerable, but people do end their lives severely demented.

In a study of some 200 elderly people with dementia dying in Belgian nursing homes, the majority were rated during the last month of their life as either severely (28%) or very severely demented (54%) (Vandervoort et al, 2013). Nearly all had continuing contact with their family, but despite remaining in touch to their death, their quality of life was judged extremely poor during those last weeks. Agitation, anxiety and fear were commonly reported by the care team, as was resistance to care, while most were reported to have experienced faecal incontinence, some degree of cachexia, difficulties with swallowing and evident pain (Vandervoort et al, 2013, pp 490-1). Despite this, family carers remain ambivalent about what they would like to see done to help: some follow a 'palliative care' model, accepting death and resisting active attempts by staff to keep their partner or parent alive, while others fear that formal carers too easily give up caring about their relative, as if once they are deemed 'too old', they are eager to disinvest in care and simply 'pull the plug' (cited in Davies et al, 2014, p 924). These narratives illustrate the 'liminality' of the fourth age – torn between the desire for a valued and valuable later life and the horror and disgust at the way long lives may end (Nicholson et al, 2012).

While the representatives of formal care, the dementia and palliative care experts have their own 'professional views' of 'good' end stage dementia care, and that expertise is fashioned out of clinical disease paradigms that assert the autonomy of the professional in determining what is 'good' (Lee et al, 2015). This includes consulting with informal carers, of course, but arguably this only envelops further those family carers within the professional standards of formal care, subordinating their agency to the superordinate structures of professional care (Raymond et al, 2014). Whatever wishes or desires the person with dementia may once have had or expressed become submerged within the policies of the various care settings or are seen as the terminal symptoms of a terminal disease. What are consequently left behind are the concerns of those who are still alive, still agentic, still asserting their identities as bereaved, skilled carers, or compassionate clinicians.

The status of personhood is harder to sustain when the person whose personhood is at issue can no longer advance or realise their identity. To argue, as Kitwood and others have done, that personhood is the essence of caring for people with dementia implies that personhood is held 'between' persons: not by one person for another (I hold her personhood for her), but as a status necessarily co-constructed by agents, by social beings. But, as we have tried to show, the problem with dementia, more than with most other 'chronic conditions' affecting older people, is that it undermines the corporeal basis for asserting agency, narrating and negotiating identity and co-constructing social relationships. If allowed to run its course, it ends with a relationship of one – the remaining agent, the agency-attributing, identity-asserting carer, looking after the orphaned body of the person with dementia. Should carers (both formal care workers and caring family members) take on that responsibility? What of the person, the person with end stage dementia who once was? Does their historical self have no role to play in this situation?

Advance care and the ownership of the self

Since entry into the state of dementia does not per se cancel agency, undermine capacity or necessarily obliterate identity, is it important for a person at the start of such a journey to exercise his or her present agency to determine his or her future care? Might they wish not to be placed in this abject relationship of one? In states where assisted suicide or voluntary euthanasia is not seen as a criminal act, this kind of question has been posed concerning the general validity of advance directives, and, more critically, of advance directives requesting voluntary euthanasia if the person reaches the point of losing all capacity and with it the power of reflexive agency (Weidemann, 2012). In this last section we try to address this most complex of all questions – namely, the extent to which present persons can exercise care over their future self.

There are two opposing positions in these kinds of debate. One is based on the concept of 'precedent autonomy' which states that 'inherent in the right to autonomy is that one's wishes be respected'; the other asserts that in the process of becoming demented 'one identity is lost and another emerges [and] it is the second person's (that is, the incompetent self's) wishes that deserve respect' (Weidemann, 2012, p 85). Weidemann poses these questions and outlines the different perspectives taken, but ultimately comes to the equivocal conclusion that 'it depends', that advance directives in general might be right in some circumstances, but not necessarily in others. She does not offer any set of rules by which one might determine when and how one or the other outcome might be the 'right' decision, although she does raise the question of whether or not the person with dementia should be deemed 'incapable' of making any 'medical' decision over his or her care.

Dutch law permits a physician to act according to advance directives, including those that request euthanasia if the patient becomes incompetent, providing that the request was voluntary, the suffering of the patient was unbearable, that another physician agrees with the course of action, that the patient was informed about his/her situation, and that together with the physician is convinced there is no reasonable alternative (van Delden, 2004, p 447). Despite this, acting on such past requests is uncommon as it requires the physician to kill the person once they can no longer make 'reasonable decisions', and that respecting patient autonomy 'does not imply that someone else is obligated to act according to [his or her] wishes' (van Delden, 2004, p 450). Other Dutch research suggests that the worlds of ethics and of professional practice rarely coincide, particularly in situations involving people with dementia, and that despite the validity assigned to the principle of 'precedent autonomy', in practice, few professionals follow through on such advance directives of people with dementia because of their very incompetence – that is, their vulnerability – at the time when action was called for (de Boer et al, 2010). Nevertheless, in one study of deaths in 594 nursing homes in Flanders, Belgium (where similar laws over assisted suicide and voluntary euthanasia apply), out of 78 cases where advance directives had been made, in only four cases, euthanasia (administration of a lethal drug with the explicit request of the resident) was performed (Vandervoort et al, 2012a).

Hertogh has argued that rather than consider the problem in terms of such deontological principles as 'precedent autonomy', it is necessary to bear in mind that 'that vulnerable persons often change their minds, particularly when their minds have changed', and that consequently a strategy of 'best interests' of the person at the time should normally apply (Hertogh, 2011, p 513). Rather than promoting the use of such advance directives, it is preferable to maintain throughout a person's care a continuing dialogue about 'advance care planning' that adapts its narrative to changing circumstances. By this there needs to be an assumption that others rather than the person with dementia increasingly represent his or her 'best interests', such that the kind of 'terminal' care practices provided reflect the views of family, friends and the staff charged with responsibility for providing care.

This immediately raises two related questions – one concerning the limits to any such co-constructed advance care planning, the other the question of whose interests are best served by any such terminal care practices. Research has begun to establish a baseline of empirical evidence of the continuing capacity of people with dementia to contribute to advance care planning. Such studies have value beyond the field of dementia, since they illustrate the possibility for all older people suffering from increasing infirmity (but who remain more or less mentally firm) and who have become reliant on the care practices of care workers to retain agency and influence over their care. It is the assumption in law that all mentally competent people have the right not to receive care or not be subject to procedures and practices that they do not wish to receive, and that those who nevertheless carry out such procedures or practices despite this are guilty of battery, but in the absence of competence and any clearly stated advance directives, no such charges can be made. The law considers the self as having conditional ownership rights over its body subject to the test of fitness to exercise such ownership rights. This is the issue of capacity, a legal concept resting equally on empirical evidence and metaphysical or moral judgement, the latter caught up with our collective social imaginaries.

Various studies have been published over the last two decades exploring this issue; to some extent it seems that while people with mild dementia can understand and make decisions about some aspects of medical care at the end of life and their likely consequences (for example, over 'do-not-resuscitate' orders, the use/non-use of tube feeding, antibiotics, blood transfusions, etc) there is little evidence that people with advanced or severe dementia can or do (Allen et al, 2003). Family members seem to be willing to contribute to such advance care planning but less as 'proxies' representing the person with dementia than as interested parties themselves, sharing in but not taking on the 'personal' view as if of the person being cared for (Hirschman et al, 2007). Studies of everyday clinical practice suggest that issues of capacity to make broad decisions about care (for example, whether or not a person with dementia can manage at home or not) often elicit disparate views among professionals. Judgements of a person's best interests tend to overshadow considerations of 'capacity' which are not often carried out unless there is some conflict within the team itself (Poole et al, 2014).

Given the likelihood that ending up in a nursing home is a decision that is rarely taken personally, a decision taken by a 'pure' agent, without consideration of the complex negotiations conducted with family members, neighbours, various medical and social care professionals, it seems unlikely that any kind of co-constructed care can be realised through the operation of an equal agency in the case of persons with dementia. The need for care in such cases reflects an incapacity to care for oneself, and that incapacity to care for oneself means that others take over some or all of the decisions that constitute care – leaving the time spent not being cared for the only space for personal agency to be expressed. If during such times the person dozes or sleeps or sits without engaging in conversation or simply passively enjoys a book, TV or music, it becomes hard for observers to confer agency or identity even if such a person's state may be understood nevertheless as 'contentment'. Only when the person cries out, interferes with others or acts in an uncivilised manner does care return – usually to put a stop to what might generally be considered undignified or uncivilised behaviour (Gilleard and Higgs, 2000). The nursing home is busy with care, but the residents are not, and at the end of the day, as much as at the end of a life, the lives of residents are circumscribed by a search for comfort and contentment rather than the pursuit of one another's interests.

Where once the elderly frail inmates of the workhouse infirmary were left to their own devices after they were locked in for the night, such neglect is rarely seen; care is continuous, to the end. Palliative care is becoming an expected part of that pathway as a way of ensuring that these old lives end without unnecessary suffering, not so much a co-constructed as a managed ending, offering as much dignity as can be afforded to those who have outlived their agency and their identity. Still they remain, for most of those who care for and about them, persons to the end, even if for most of us still exercising agency and seeking to realise our identities as the not yet so old, it is an ending for which we have little interest and even less desire to plan for (Price et al, 2014).

Conclusions

The ending of any life is tragic, whether the death of a still-born baby who will never have the chance to develop his or her 'personhood' or of an old and very demented person whose chances to negotiate his or her personhood have long since been lost. In considering care at the limits of human experience, particularly that care associated with advanced dementia, we have sought to address several related issues – whether or not it is meaningful to treat people in such circumstances as having 'lost' their personhood, and if we do, whether that means we should care any the less for or about them, and if we should not cease to care or to care less, whether we must care differently and if so, how? Our position throughout has been that personhood is best conceived as a status and not as a corporeal or psychic phenomenon, and that it is generally better to think of people as expressing agency, articulating identity, as well as having or failing to have that agency and identity acknowledged within the practices of care. Personhood in this sense is negotiated, as a status, between persons. It does not confer any inherent rights beyond those due to all human beings however impaired – that is, human rights. The ability to exercise rights – such as the ability to shape an individual's personhood status – depends not just on other persons but on the existence of a number of cognitive and corporeal capacities. Most people who reach an advanced stage of dementia, we have argued, retain few such capacities, and those that are retained are relatively ineffectual when it comes to negotiating one's personhood status. An individual's identity as a human being, a person, may be indisputable, but his or her capacity to realise his or her rights can be so compromised that these rights exist only in so far as they are attributed by society to each and every human being – such as the right not to be hurt, harmed or humiliated. Under such circumstances it could be argued that it is the carers who can best realise these rights, through their recognition and their reflexivity, as it is embodied in their actively carrying out the various caregiving tasks that seem most in the interest of the person they care for; in short, through their actions as moral agents. Realising these interests, however, may not automatically over-ride the interests of others – those of the carer, their colleagues, their family and those of the other residents – no matter how disabled the person may be. For carers, particularly, choices have to be made.

Few people enter the labour force as 'a carer' without some desire to be of help to others, to do a good job and at the same time receive due rewards. The care relationship between parents and children, between partners, or between friends is different from the care relationship in both domiciliary and residential long-term care. Of course there are points of similarity, and formal care can both complement and substitute for the tasks of informal caring. But a distinction can be made between emotional labour and acts determined by love or affinity (Hochschild, 2003). The demand that carers express and promote any particular feeling for the person they care for is consequently unreasonable and, we would argue, counter-productive. This does not mean that carers have no feelings, and nor does it mean that they never develop any feelings for those for whom they care. But such feelings should not be part of anyone's job description or professional qualifications. Not to feel pity for people with severe or end stage illnesses with whom the carer is working would seem to be unusual, worrying, perhaps, to both the carer, his or her colleagues and any friends or relatives still in close contact with the person being cared for. But pity, as we have tried to show, is a response to another's misfortune; it is not a necessary part of any person's job.

The move towards palliative care for people with dementia raises many more issues than those associated with traditional dementia care where the focus understandably has been on minimising abjection and reinforcing identity, facilitating as much agency as the person can still express, and preventing as far as is possible any unnecessary suffering. As we have written, in residential and domiciliary care settings those concerns will still need to be balanced with other equally valid interests, both in terms of employment and in terms of the worker's own identity. Perhaps caring at the limits is in the end easier because it requires no negotiation and no dialectic. But it is hardly any less painful or any less tragic to witness what is not just an ending but a failure both of life and of the hope embodied in care. In the end it might be wisest to simply echo Beckett's words, to 'fail better' and make of that what we will.

NINE

Conclusion

Whatever the balance between successful and unsuccessful ageing that is achieved by a particular generation or society, each success creates in its shadow new possibilities of failure. As more people age there are more examples, of both success and failure. The presence of the unsuccessfully aged, whether framed as the 'aged and infirm' or as those 'impotent through age' sees them become the objects of what we have called society's moral imperative of care. Where once their numbers were few and their circumstances more amenable to resolution, in contemporary ageing societies their predicament has become more challenging as the later lives of successive cohorts have improved. In response, the post-war welfare state has searched for alternative 'postmodern' resolutions beyond the modern developments of pensions and long-stay hospital beds. Community care, deinstitutionalisation and the marketisation of services have all been adopted and all found wanting.

Even in the light of scandals, funding crises and market failures, the moral imperative of care remains unchallenged. The provision of care for aged and infirm persons, now especially including those with mental infirmity, has lost none of its ethical underpinnings. Arguably it has become more sensitive to quality of life concerns compared with the care regimes of first modernity. This is reflected in the centrality of terms such as 'dignity' and 'person-centred care' in motivating improvement in the provision of formal care. In this book we have approached the problem of 'unsuccessful' ageing through the rubric of the fourth age and its positioning within the moral imperative of care. In particular we have considered how the new vocabulary of 'personhood' and 'person-centred' care serves to reduce the impact of such failure.

Personhood has become a pivotal term among those concerned with improving care particularly for people with dementia. Acknowledging the importance of personhood has become one of the defining aspects of policy and practice in dementia care (NICE, 2006; Nuffield Council on Bioethics, 2009; Thomas and Milligan, 2015). A concern for person-centred care is not confined to those working in this area, and has been applied more generally to people of all ages, and with varied disabilities and impairments. What makes the articulation of these arguments within the field of dementia care so significant is the way that dementia itself has been understood. Dementia – or major neurocognitive disorder, as it is now termed in DSM-V (*Diagnostic and Statistical Manual of Mental Disorders*, 5th edn) – by definition seems to represent the loss of identity and self-hood, with some writers viewing dementia as 'the loss of self' (Cohen and Eisdorfer, 2001) or 'the loss of the person' (Sweeting and Gilhooly, 1997).

This perspective has been challenged on two grounds: first, that it exaggerates the extent of deficits experienced by people who develop dementia, and second, that it misrepresents what a person or 'personhood' really is (Kitwood, 1993, 1997b; Downs, 1997). In a number of works, Tom Kitwood outlined what he saw as the fundamental denial of personhood in many care settings for people with dementia (Kitwood, 1993, 1997a; Kitwood and Bredin, 1992). Under the influence of the extreme individualism that Kitwood believed was dominating Western societies, personhood was being reduced to two criteria: autonomy and rationality (Kitwood, 1997a, p 9). This reduction of personhood to such an individualised conception of cognitive competence, he argued, has profound implications for the moral recognition of people with mental impairments. As a counter to this, Kitwood contended that personhood should be conceptualised more broadly, where relationships and moral solidarity are its foundational principles, in order to overcome 'a social psychology that is malignant in its effects' (Kitwood, 1997a, p 14).

In this book we have argued that personhood is a polysemous construct that confounds morality with metaphysics. It could be argued that thinking and talking of persons is part of everyday language, signifying little more than its surface level, meaning an individual, a person, a 'someone', etc. However, within policy and professional practice personhood is used to convey more than this 'everyday' meaning; it forms an important signifier in what might be thought of as the new semiotics of care. The failure to treat persons with dementia as persons, it is claimed, is not only undesirable, but is itself a source of further problematising, if not the progressing, of dementia. Hence the use of terms such as 'malign positioning' or a 'malign social psychology' in writings advocating person-centred care (Kitwood, 1997a; Sabat, 2006). Indeed, Tom Kitwood had argued that by replacing a malignant social psychology with a benign and supportive 'dementia culture' it might be possible for at least some older people to become 'remented' – by which he seemed to mean restored to the state they were in before the onset of dementia (Kitwood and Bredin, 1992; Sixsmith et al, 1993).

In interrogating the concept of personhood, we first separated the metaphysical underpinnings of personhood from its status as a moral category. We then explored the distinction between philosophical and social scientific understanding of the term. As regards the former, we concluded that personhood considered as a moral category offered little additional purchase beyond that conveyed by the status of human being (Higgs and Gilleard, 2016). In its metaphysical incarnation, personhood can be understood as an omnibus term made up of distinct elements – such as agency, reflexive consciousness, personal identity, memory and rationality – each of which can be explored through analytical as well as empirical research (see, for example, Rorty, 1975; Howorth and Saper, 2003; Clare et al, 2005; Fazio and Mitchell, 2009). As regards the social sciences, they have had at best an agnostic view of the self and the construct of personhood, which tend to be treated as similar or equivalent terms. What most writers in this tradition have recognised is the difficulty in separating the social from the personal. Durkheim used the term '*homo duplex*' as a way of recognising that however social the construct of 'person' or 'self' might be, the social alone cannot adequately account for the totality contained by these terms. While persons cannot exist as persons outside the context of society, it is equally true that human society cannot exist without the engagement of humans as distinct corporeal beings. While the wilder fringes of social constructionism might see persons as no more than discursive articulations, nodal points in a web of social relationships possessing neither agency nor authorial identity, a certain degree of conscious corporeality seems necessary for there to be something by which to embody personhood.

Care is more unequivocally social. Yet it, too, cannot be realised by discourse alone; it requires some form of social practice that is embedded in particular social relations. Care 'recognises' but does not 'realise' persons; rather, it represents the realisation of particular forms of social relationship that in the present day take the form of kinship or contract. Ambivalence pervades both such forms of care, which is itself never wholly benign, hence its connection to the social imaginary of the fourth age. Whether familial or contractual, care cannot take a disinterested approach to the recipient of such care, nor can the recipient of care fail to acknowledge the person providing it. But carer and cared for are neither interchangeable persons, nor are they interchangeable roles. While reciprocity and the co-construction of identity within the care relationship might be evident during the early stages of familial care, such as that between a married couple, where one partner begins showing signs of increasing dependency, the general direction of travel is of a growing one-sidedness in the relationship, towards what might be called 'a relationship of one'. Studies have observed how family members often experience increasing feelings of 'loss' as their relative's dementia progresses – whether the loss of companionship, of a shared past or indeed of a common future (Gillies, 2012; Førsund et al, 2015). In compensation for such experiences, increased effort is required from informal carers to maintain meaning and continuity in the relationship (Hellstrom et al, 2007; McGovern, 2011; Shim et al, 2013), in effect, exercising a kind of 'authorial control' over the nature of the relationship. Obviously within formal care settings, particularly in the context of the nursing home, carers' behaviour is determined by their contractual role – and care is constructed in part as a set of duties and practices determined by management, and in part by their perceptions of the residents' needs. Given the absence of a shared past and of elaborate, co-constructed identities, what forms the material of their caring relationship is at best, to adapt Clifford Geertz's term, a 'thin' identity, constructed through and by the older person's frailty and by recorded biographical details, aka 'the history' (Geertz, 1994).

Such formally constructed relationships share certain features – their one-sidedness, their ahistoricity and their limited capacity for 'co-constructing' the present within the context of the past. This is not just a matter of differential power such as that existing between prison warders and prisoners or between nurses and their patients. In cases of dementia and other forms of severe cognitive impairment, there exists 'an incapacity of the mind' that limits the expression of some key components of personhood, most notably those of agency, autonomy and reflexivity, which allow a person to represent him or herself to the other as a particular person or self. This does not mean that people with major cognitive impairments are simply passive objects of care, lacking desires, feelings and intentions. Behind many of the conflicts of care and much of the abuse within it lies a clash of wills, a desire not to be cared for, or feelings of anger or fear, albeit these are not always coherently articulated. Nor is any of this constant: there is a degree of variability that undermines the possibility for any strategy of care to be consistently adopted, to enable care to be carried out by rule alone. Care requires constant adaptation – by the carers – which is no doubt why more experienced care workers are less likely to be subject to being struck or abused than those with more limited experience.

As Rodriquez has pointed out, attributions of agency toward residents made by care staff reflect judgements based less on empirical evidence than on the meaning-making of the staff – who tend to credit agency for valued actions and outcomes and deny it for what is (by them) undesired or undesirable (Rodriquez, 2014). Formal carers embody the moral imperative of care. They act as moral agents, and as such they confer moral identities on each other, as well as on family members and on the residents themselves. The practices of care as well as the practitioners are themselves given moral status as the embodiment of that imperative. But, although conferring moral status, caregiving tasks also represent dirty work, embodying the position of the carer as well as the abjection of the persons they care for. Protection against the ignominy of the fourth age necessarily invokes it – symbolised, for example, by use of adult diapers/nappies or incontinence pads. The dignity that is invoked by the moral imperative to care does not transcend the nature of the tasks involved in carrying it out. Neither does it remove the stain of abjection that is attached to the person being cared for, even though it may valorise the moral agency of the carer. While both carer and cared for are human beings within the framework of the care relationship, this does not confer a moral equivalence. This non-equivalence is also true in the case of respect and agency. While informal care is dependent on maintaining a 'thick' relationship, it is more vulnerable to its collapse. Formal care breaks down only in circumstances of the contract, not the care relationship as such, as it rests on a 'thinner' but more flexible underpinning.

Personhood and a critique of the philosophy of care

Sustaining a thin version of personhood in circumstances of the fourth age may have virtues but it has a limited capacity to serve as a 'philosophy of care'. Interrogating the notion of personhood and its relationship to dementia we sought to make clear how much more complex the concept is than it appears at first viewing. Kitwood's assumptions about personhood, we have argued, confound metaphysical with moral philosophy, while leaving open the prospect that the only conditions threatening adult personhood are those that arise when the circumstances of dementia are transformed by a 'malignant' social psychology. By taking the position that personhood is an attribute of relationships, not capabilities, Kitwood sidestepped consideration of what could be termed the 'component approach' to personhood, those necessary and sufficient conditions that render personhood possible, all the while treating social relationships as if not potentially identical, at least potentially equivalent.

Kitwood confounded the constitution of personhood with the conditions for its existence; namely, that it exists in an 'I-thou' relationship, the responsibility for which, although unspecified, seems implicitly to be that of the carer's. By avoiding further considerations of personhood, Kitwood ended up treating personhood as little more than a moral entity, 'a valid object of our moral concern' (Ohlin, 2005, p 237), and as such, deserving those rights that follow from being of 'moral concern' without further questions or qualification. While we have no dispute with recognising that people with dementia are and should be objects of moral concern, as indeed should all human beings, whatever their disabilities, we also recognise that many people with dementia lack some of the capabilities deemed to constitute metaphysical personhood – such as self-awareness, reflexivity, second-order volition and narrative unity – and that such deficits increase with time. The problems with a personhood-centred approach to helping people with such impairments are twofold. In the first place, Kitwood's approach fails to distinguish between maintaining the moral standing of persons and preserving their capabilities of performing personhood. The failure to recognise this distinction places the burden of responsibility on other persons for sustaining the personhood of individuals with dementia, not just in the sense of sustaining moral concern for them, but also in preserving their capabilities for personhood. The failure to achieve the former is too easily treated as a failure to realise the latter, and the blame placed in the hands of the carer.

Second, as others have noted, Kitwood's original conceptualisation of personhood was rooted in a Christian theological assumption in which all humans have intrinsic worth. His later work abandoned this religious underpinning, leaving it less coherent and more relativist (Baldwin and Capstick, 2007, p 180). Instead of using personhood as a 'superfluous, confusing and without pragmatic use' term 'that can be easily used as a cover-up concept' (Gordijn, 1999, p 356) to improve the position of people with dementia, we would argue that it is better to avoid the term in professional and policy discourse while recognising its utility in everyday language.

It is necessary to acknowledge at this point that there is a non-equivalence in both the moral status of carers and the cared for, and in their relative capacity for articulating agency and for eliciting reciprocity. In this latter sense, it is the responsibility of the carer to treat the people they care for with respect, to safeguard their interests and identities, and to be responsive to their needs and feelings. Doing so deserves public regard in a way that being given a diagnosis of dementia does not: by this we do not mean that people with dementia are lesser beings or that they should not receive due care and concern. Carers can act as moral agents, while people with severe dementia (that is, the people who are looked after by formal paid carers) cannot.

Valuing the former does not imply devaluing the latter. What matters is recognising the agency of carers, particularly their activation of what Harry Frankfurt has termed their 'second-order motives', not to do what at times they may feel like doing, not hitting back, not shouting back, not turning away from the more ugly aspects of care, as well as their rationality and reflexivity in thinking round the problems and puzzles of care.

Formal care can be viewed as both a job and a duty; the capacity to carry out the various tasks of care while maintaining a social relationship with the person being looked after is frequently demanding. However, to call on a philosophy of care that privileges a particular interpretation of personhood is as likely to confound as it is to clarify what should or what should not be done, as well as what can and what cannot be done. An alternative approach is to see dementia care in terms of containing and contesting the malign *social imaginary* of the fourth age that particularly surrounds formal care (Gilleard and Higgs, 2010; Higgs and Gilleard, 2015). We have deliberately chosen this terminology so as to contrast it with Kitwood's phrase 'malignant *social psychology*' (or indeed Sabat's 2006 'malignant *positioning*') because both these latter formulations stress inter-personal rather than social processes. This does not mean neglecting the study of individual agency, of memory, of narrative identity, or of a sense of self in people with dementia, and neither does it mean abandoning attempts to support people's existing capabilities while minimising the harmful consequences of their incapacities. Most carers, paid as well as unpaid, can and do recognise the moral standing of people with dementia and respond through what we have identified as a moral imperative of care. Despite this, their care practices may either deepen or lighten the darkness of the fourth age. To consider how to minimise contributing to the former and to maximise the latter, we suggest, requires no moral or metaphysical assertions about the 'personhood' of people with dementia beyond those associated with the recognition of a common humanity and the taking of due care.

What might a 'philosophy of care' informed by a 'fourth age' perspective look like? Arguably it would eschew any such philosophy *qua* philosophy, considering, instead, the factors influencing the practices of informal and formal care and the relative constraints on 'doing otherwise' in the sense of helping carers avoid doing too little or too much for the person they care for, all the while supporting their meaning-making in enabling as decent a life as possible for the person for whom they are caring. At an abstract level this could be construed as equally supporting the moral and the metaphysical elements of personhood of the carer, supporting them to care rationally and reflexively considering what is in the best interests of the individual, and with a sense of compassion or pity for their infirmity, abjection, dependency and loss. However, as we have pointed out, such an abstract elaboration is not necessarily called for in order to reach these objectives.

As 'dementia care' seems to become the dominant paradigm of late life care, the dilemmas faced by people looking after older people with dementia may, as a consequence, be too readily generalised to older people whose infirmity is not the consequence of major cognitive impairment. While the responsibility for looking after someone with dementia often invokes a relationship of one, this necessary one-sidedness can also be too easily applied to other infirm older people whose failures are of a different sort – of sensory impairment, skeletal-muscular weakness or degenerative disease – that have less impact on the structures underlying the metaphysical components of personhood. Older infirm people who assert their own agency, identity and desires may be seen to be as difficult to care for as people with dementia, whether because of their physical immobility and as a result of their difficulties transferring or using the toilet, or because of their refusal to share in the co-construction of the care relationship by others, for example, by 'over' or 'under' estimating their need for care. Assuming agency, rationality and reciprocity from the person being cared for under such circumstances might constitute less an unreasonable set of demands generated by the carers on a person unable to rise to them than a reasonable strategy to avoid activating a fourth age imaginary. While the *selective* withholding of attributions of agency when caring for people with dementia may prove a way of coping without 'blaming' the person – for example, for reacting aggressively to attempts at care – generalising this to people who simply choose to resist the ministrations of care might lead to less positive outcomes. Is there then a risk that in the care for people with dementia, successful care practices selectively invoke a fourth age imaginary, to maintain the person's moral identity, while the very opposite is the case when caring for older people whose infirmity does not extend to their mental functioning? In the final section of this chapter we consider such possibilities.

The fourth age imaginary: aid or obstacle to care?

In our book, *Rethinking old age: Theorising the fourth age*, we outlined the different elements constituting its social imaginary. We contrasted its status as an imaginary with that of the third age that we have represented as a cultural field. The intention behind this was to acknowledge a major point of fracture in later life, between the 'cultures of ageing' and the fears of a 'residualised' old age. In our argument there was little positive about the feared imaginary of the fourth age; it was not a position to be desired, nor was it to be contemplated as a potentially meaningful, 'transgressive' position. While we would not disagree in general terms with this formulation, our consideration in relation to the issue of personhood and care in advanced old age is formulated around the question of whether or not there may not be some other meaning to be made out of this imaginary.

Several writers (including Kitwood) have castigated the emphasis on rationality within our 'hyper-cognitive' individualistic culture (Kitwood, 1997a; Post, 1995, 2006). In opposing this position, there has been a call to recognise a common humanity and a shared vulnerability, and to advocate an alternative culture that privileges 'relatedness' over 'rationality' (Kitwood and Benson, 1995). The assumption seems to be that unless we find a way to 'include' or 'maintain' people with dementia in everyday life, the danger is that they will suffer the ignominy of exclusion and social death. In place of an emphasis on agency, intent and planning, such writers wish to privilege feelings and relatedness – which they assume exist either in some separate compartment of the brain or in some other form of social relationship.

Earlier, we raised the distinction between care of those who are mentally infirm and those whose infirmity is primarily physical in nature. We suggested that while resistance to the attributions of a fourth age imaginary was obviously beneficial for the latter group, it might prove deleterious at least in some circumstances for those with major cognitive impairment, putting the individual at risk not just of physical harm but of further abjection and greater indignity. While we would not argue that people with mild or moderate degrees of cognitive impairment lack any agency, intentions or desires, we would also posit that in the late stages of dementia, intentionality may not be just simply difficult to discern, but could, in fact, dissolve into a state of being that exists without a corresponding desire to assert or express any particular identity or to realise any particular style or quality of life. At the extremities of old age, there may be an end to wanting, an end to wanting responsibilities, an end to needing to express oneself, and an end, even, to wanting to be someone. In such circumstances might the fourth age be a sort of haven from such striving and an escape from the weight of failed choices?

At all stages caring for others remains a social relationship. This relationship is only at the most abstract level one of equality. The greater the infirmity, the deeper the abjection, the more limited the mental capacities of the person being cared for, the more responsibility for shaping that relationship comes to rest with the person providing care and his or her intentions and understanding. Interpretations by carers of 'best interests' must hold more weight than the expressions of an autonomy that can at best only be interpreted. What constitutes best interests are, at least in part, the product of the various cultures of the service organisation, the family and of wider society. Recognising the pervasiveness of the fourth age social imaginary, and when it can and cannot be resisted, forms part of what constitutes caregivers' experience and expertise. This is often not recognised when the emphasis is placed on the discourses or professional ethics surrounding the personhood of the cared for individual, effectively ignoring or subordinating the personhood of the carer.

Carers themselves may be equally, if differently, 'infirm', and equally, if differently, at risk of becoming 'abject'. Their identity and agency too may be constrained – in the case of formal carers, by the demands of 'management' or of 'relatives', and in the case of informal carers, by other family members and service providers. And, of course, there are some people with chronic conditions and progressive disabilities, particularly those with early onset dementia, whose appearance is not consonant with the corporeal markers of 'real' old age and whose advocacy and activities embody both agency, 'citizenship' and identity. Such exceptions may seem to prove the rule, but they also risk seeking to contradict one imaginary with another that is arguably more fragile, more tenuous and less easily sustained.

Conclusions

We have argued in this book that the moral imperative of care forms an essential part of, and helps realise, the fourth age as a social presence in people's lives. The idea of personhood is connected to the fourth age in terms of its imputed role in combating frailty and abjection, which emerges through a renewed and reformulated moral imperative of care. Personhood, however, is not as straightforward a term as might seem. It draws on two rather different types of meaning: one concerned with what constitutes the basis for each human being's unique individuality and the other on the shared moral (or legal) status that human beings possess. In the sense of the former, of what might be called the self or personal identity, age-associated mental infirmity, Alzheimer's disease or major cognitive impairment presents a distinct challenge to that individuality, both in its expression and in its recognition. The major cognitive impairment that negatively defines people with dementia affects their communication, experience and understanding. Although this is obviously a matter of degree and varies over time and between people, the progress of such impairment provides a growing challenge to the individual's capacity to realise the 'components' of personhood. This is equally true for those caring for people with dementia. They, too, face difficulties in maintaining their agency, their identity and their status as persons, as well as in their attempts to help sustain and support their dependent's personal agency and identity.

For different reasons, the problem of dementia also has an impact on an individual's moral status or rather, on their moral equivalence. Moral status can be used in two different and distinct ways, as either moral agency or moral identity (or standing). Moral agency is invoked when questions of responsibility and accountability are at issue. Moral identity, by contrast, refers to entitlements or rights. Thus it can be argued that not everyone possesses the same moral agency (most notably in the case of the legal position of the mentally ill or mentally incompetent), while arguing that every human being possesses the same rights or entitlements. While differences in moral agency were once used to calibrate a person's moral identity (or standing), such as someone who is judged as not competent to plead in court, sign legal documents or make judgements concerning their personal affairs, increasingly this merging of categories (between identity and agency) has been challenged. This has seen the emergence in national, supra-national and global organisations of a commitment to forms of universal human rights. This has been taken up by advocates for mentally ill and intellectually handicapped people, and more recently by advocates of people with dementia.

While we have no difficulty with the arguments put forward by those demanding that the rights of social citizenship be extended to people with dementia, including their participation in policy and practice (Bartlett and O'Connor, 2010), we also acknowledge that people with dementia may also, and not unreasonably, be judged to 'lack capacity' to manage their own affairs. The cover provided by the use of the personhood discourse risks concealing such critical distinctions, both in terms of its articulation as a moral status and as a metaphysical construct. We are still faced with the problems of care in both their moral and practical sense. While it can be argued that persons not lacking capacity (whatever their diagnostic status) must be free to negotiate (and hence co-construct) their care, whether within the moral and social framework of the family or within the framework of formally contracted care, the dilemmas of caring for those lacking capacity (in some form or another) are harder to resolve. The social citizenship evoked by Alzheimer's advocates and activists may not lighten those particular shadows; indeed, it may only darken them further, compounding their existing difficulties with a further failure to 'live well' with dementia.

While we have criticised those who attribute a kind of 'quasi' agency to people with evident incapacities, we would also reject the position of those such as Peter Singer (1993), who argue that people limited by major cognitive impairments have less entitlement to call on resources than others with unimpaired rationality and full capacity for self-awareness. Rather than risking the slippery discourse of personhood, we have argued for the relevance of the concept of a 'fourth age imaginary'. This imaginary of old age identifies its social and cultural moorings while simultaneously recognising its intimate connection to the moral imperative of care. In itself, such recognition will not solve the problems of care. What we have tried to show is how the discourses of the fourth age necessarily imbricate the practices of care and shape their understanding. These can be at some moments contradictory and at other times complementary. Certain aspects or practices of care can risk bringing down the fourth age on to the individual by denying them agency, identity or personal suffering, just as other practices may serve to protect people from its abjection and failure. Insisting on the need to consistently choose one over the other may not necessarily be the best for either the person being cared for or for the carer. Sometimes care itself may need its haven.

References

Aalten, P., de Vugt, M.E., Jaspers, N., Jolles, J. and Verhey, F.R. (2005) 'The course of neuropsychiatric symptoms in dementia. Part I: findings from the two-year longitudinal Maasbed study', *International Journal of Geriatric Psychiatry*, 20, 6, 523-30.

Ablitt, A., Jones, G.V. and Muers, J. (2009) 'Living with dementia: A systematic review of the influence of relationship factors', *Aging & Mental Health*, 13, 4, 497-511.

Abrahamson, K., Suitor, J.J. and Pillemer, K. (2009) 'Conflict between nursing home staff and residents' families does it increase burnout?', *Journal of Aging and Health*, 21, 6, 895-912.

Adams, K.B. (2006) 'The transition to caregiving: the experience of family members embarking on the dementia caregiving career', *Journal of Gerontological Social Work*, 47, 3/4, 3-29.

Adams, T. (2008) *Dementia care nursing: Promoting well-being in people with dementia and their families*, Basingstoke: Palgrave Macmillan.

Afram, B., Stephan, A., Verbeek, H., Bleijlevens, M.H.C., Suhonen, R., Sutcliffe, C. et al (2014) 'Reasons for institutionalization of people with dementia: Informal caregiver reports from 8 European countries', *Journal of the American Medical Directors Association*, 15, 108-16.

Aguero-Torres, H., von Strauss, E., Viitanen, M., Winblad, B. and Fratiglioni, L. (2001) 'Institutionalization in the elderly: the role of chronic diseases and dementia. Cross-sectional and longitudinal data from a population-based study', *Journal of Clinical Epidemiology*, 54, 6, 795-801.

Ahmad, S. and O'Mahony, M.S. (2005) 'Where older people die: a retrospective population-based study', *QJM*, 98, 12, 865-70.

Allen, R.S., DeLaine, S.R., Chaplin, W.F., Marson, D.C., Bourgeois, M.S., Dijkstra, K. et al (2010) 'Elderly persons' experiences of striving to receive care on their own terms in nursing homes', *International Journal of Nursing Practice*, 16, 1, 64-8.

Anderberg, P. and Berglund, A.L. (2010) 'Elderly persons' experiences of striving to receive care on their own terms in nursing homes', *International Journal of Nursing Practice*, 16, 1, 64-8.

Anderson, B. (2000) *Doing the dirty work: The global politics of domestic labour*, London: Zed Books.

Anderson, M. (1985) 'The emergence of the modern life cycle in Britain', *Social History*, 10, 1, 82-4.

Andersson, I., Pettersson, E. and Sidenvall, B. (2007) 'Daily life after moving into a care home – experiences from older people, relatives and contact persons', *Journal of Clinical Nursing*, 16, 9, 1712-18.

Andrew, M.K., Mitnitski, A.B. and Rockwood, K. (2008) 'Social vulnerability, frailty and mortality in elderly people', *PLoS ONE*, 3, 5, e2232, 1-8.

Archer, M.S. (1988) *Culture and agency: The place of culture in social theory*, Cambridge: Cambridge University Press.

Archer, M.S. (1995) *Realist social theory: The morphogenetic approach*, Cambridge: Cambridge University Press.

Archer, M.S. (2000) *Being human: The problem of agency*, Cambridge: Cambridge University Press.

Aronson, J. and Neysmith, S.M. (1997) 'The retreat of the state and long-term care provision: Implications for frail elderly people, unpaid family carers and paid home care workers', *Studies in Political Economy*, 53, 37-66.

Ashforth, B.E. and Kreiner, G.E. (1999) '"How can you do it?": Dirty work and the challenge of constructing a positive identity', *The Academy of Management Review*, 24, 3, 413-34.

Bäckman, L. and MacDonald, S.W. (2006) 'Death and cognition: Synthesis and outlook', *European Psychologist*, 11, 3, 224.

Bagri, A.S. and Tiberius, R. (2010) 'Medical student perspectives on geriatrics and geriatric education', *Journal of the American Geriatrics Society*, 58, 10, 1994-9.

Baker, A.A. (1975) 'Granny battering', *Modern Geriatrics*, 8, 20-4.

Baldwin, C. and Capstick, A. (2007) *Tom Kitwood on dementia: A reader and critical commentary*, Maidenhead: McGraw-Hill Education.

Ballard, C., Fossey, J., Chithramohan, R., Howard, R., Burns, A., Thompson, P. et al (2001) 'Quality of care in private sector and NHS facilities for people with dementia: cross sectional survey', *BMJ*, 323, 7310, 426-7.

Baltes, P.B. (1987) 'Theoretical propositions of life-span developmental psychology: On the dynamics between growth and decline', *Developmental Psychology*, 23, 5, 611-26.

Baltes, P.B. (2006) 'Facing our limits: Human dignity in the very old', *Daedalus*, 135, 1, 32-9.

Baltes, P.B. and Baltes, M.M. (1990) 'Psychological perspectives on successful aging: The model of selective optimization with compensation', *Successful Aging: Perspectives from the Behavioral Sciences*, 1, 1-34.

References

Baltes, P.B. and Schaie, K.W. (1976) 'On the plasticity of intelligence in adulthood and old age: Where Horn and Donaldson fail', *American Psychologist*, 31, 720-5.

Baltes, P.B. and Smith, J. (1999) 'Multilevel and systemic analyses of old age: Theoretical and empirical evidence for a fourth age', in V.L. Bengston and K.W. Schaie (eds) *Handbook of theories of aging*, New York: Springer Publishing, pp 153-73.

Baltes, P.B. and Smith, J. (2003) 'New frontiers in the future of aging: From successful aging of the young old to the dilemmas of the fourth age', *Gerontology*, 49, 2, 123-35.

Banijamali, S., Jacoby, D. and Hagopian, A. (2014) 'Characteristics of home care workers who leave their jobs: a cross-sectional study of job satisfaction and turnover in Washington state', *Home Health Care Services Quarterly*, 33, 3, 137-58.

Bartlett, R. and O'Connor, D. (2010) *Broadening the dementia debate: Toward social citizenship*, Bristol: Policy Press.

Bataille, G. (1979) 'The psychological structure of fascism' (translated by C.R. Lovitt), *New German Critique*, 16, 64-87.

Bataille, G. (1999) 'Abjection and miserable forms', in S. Lotringer (ed) *More and less*, Cambridge, MA: MIT Press, pp 8-13.

Beauchamp, T.L. (1999) 'The failure of theories of personhood', *Kennedy Institute of Ethics Journal*, 9, 4, 309-24.

Bebbington, A.C. (1979) 'Changes in the provision of social services to the elderly in the community over fourteen years', *Social Policy and Administration*, 13, 2, 111-23.

Beck, U. (2001) 'Interview with Ulrich Beck', *Journal of Consumer Culture*, 1, 2, 261-77.

Beck, U. and Beck-Gernsheim E. (2002) *Individualization. institutionalized individualism and its social and political consequences*, London: Sage.

Beck, U., Giddens, A. and Lash, S. (1994) *Reflexive modernization: Politics, tradition and aesthetics in the modern social order*, Cambridge: Polity.

Beck, U., Bonss, W. and Lau, C. (2003) 'The theory of reflexive modernisation: problematic, hypotheses and research programme', *Theory, Culture & Society*, 20, 2, 1-33.

Becker, G. (1994) 'The oldest old: Autonomy in the face of frailty', *Journal of Aging Studies*, 8, 1, 59-76.

Beckett, S. (2006) *The complete dramatic works*, London: Faber & Faber.

Belfield, C., Cribb, J., Hood, A. and Joyce, R. (2014) *Living standards, poverty and inequality in the UK: 2014*, London: Institute for Fiscal Studies.

Berdes, C. and Eckert, J.M. (2007) 'The language of caring: Nurse's aides' use of family metaphors conveys affective care', *The Gerontologist*, 47, 3, 340-9.

Bharucha, A.J., Pandav, R., Shen, C., Dodge, H.H. and Ganguli, M. (2004) 'Predictors of nursing facility admission: a 12-year epidemiological study in the United States', *Journal of the American Geriatrics Society*, 52, 3, 434-9.

Bittman, M., Matheson, G. and Meagher, G. (1999) 'The changing boundary between home and market: Australian trends in outsourcing domestic labour', *Work, Employment & Society*, 13, 2, 249-73.

Blessed, G., Tomlinson, B.E. and Roth, M. (1968) 'The association between quantitative measures of dementia and of senile change in the cerebral grey matter of elderly subjects', *The British Journal of Psychiatry*, 114, 797-811.

Block, N. (1995) 'How many concepts of consciousness?', *Behavioral and Brain Sciences*, 18, 2, 272-87.

Booth, T. (1985) *Home truths*, Aldershot: Gower.

Bortz W. (2010) 'Understanding Frailty', *The Journals of Gerontology. Series A, Biological sciences and medical sciences*, 65, 3, 255-56.

Bowers, B.J., Fibich, B. and Jacobson, N. (2001) 'Care-as-service, care-as-relating, care-as-comfort: Understanding nursing home residents' definitions of quality', *The Gerontologist*, 41, 4, 539-45.

Boyle, P.A., Buchman, A.S., Wilson, R.S., Leurgans, S.E. and Bennett, D.A. (2010) 'Physical frailty is associated with incident mild cognitive impairment in community-based older persons', *Journal of the American Geriatrics Society*, 58, 2, 248-55.

Broad, J.B., Gott, M., Kim, H., Boyd, M., Chen, H. and Connolly, M.J. (2013) 'Where do people die? An international comparison of the percentage of deaths occurring in hospital and residential aged care settings in 45 populations, using published and available statistics', *International Journal of Public Health*, 58, 2, 257-67.

Brodaty, H. and Donkin, M. (2009) 'Family caregivers of people with dementia', *Dialogues in Clinical Neuroscience*, 11, 2, 217-28.

Brodaty, H., Draper, B. and Low, L.F. (2003) 'Nursing home staff attitudes towards residents with dementia: strain and satisfaction with work', *Journal of Advanced Nursing*, 44, 6, 583-90.

Brownie, S. and Nancarrow, S. (2013) 'Effects of person-centered care on residents and staff in aged-care facilities: a systematic review', *Clinical Interventions in Aging*, 8, 1-10.

Bryden, C. (2015) *Nothing about us, without us! 20 years of dementia advocacy*, London: Jessica Kingsley Publishers.

Bubeck, D.E. (1995) *Care, gender and justice*, Oxford: Clarendon Press.

Buchman, A.S., Boyle, P.A., Wilson, R.S., Tang, Y. and Bennett, D.A. (2007) 'Frailty is associated with incident Alzheimer's disease and cognitive decline in the elderly', *Psychosomatic Medicine*, 69, 5, 483-9.

Burkitt, P. (1991) *Social selves*, London: Sage Publications.

Burrow, J.A. (1986) *Ages of man: A study in medieval writing and thought*, Oxford: Clarendon Press.

Bursto, G.R. (1975) 'Granny bashing (letter)', *British Medical Journal*, 3, 592.

Burton, A.M., Sautter, J.M., Tulsky, J.A., Lindquist, J.H., Hays, J.C., Olsen, M.K. et al (2012) 'Burden and well-being among a diverse sample of cancer, congestive heart failure, and chronic obstructive pulmonary disease caregivers', *Journal of Pain and Symptom Management*, 44, 3, 410-20.

Bury, M. (1982) 'Chronic illness as biographical disruption', *Sociology of Health & Illness*, 4, 167-82.

Caetano, A. (2015) 'Defining personal reflexivity A critical reading of Archer's approach', *European Journal of Social Theory*, 18, 1, 60-75.

Callegaro, F. (2012) 'The ideal of the person: Recovering the novelty of Durkheim's sociology. Part 1: The idea of society and its relation to the individual', *Journal of Classical Sociology*, 12, 3-4, 449-78.

Carrithers, M. (1985) 'An alternative social history of the self', in M. Carrithers, S. Collins and S. Lukes (eds) (1985) *The category of the person: Anthropology, philosophy, history*, Cambridge: Cambridge University Press, pp 234-56.

Carruth, A.K., Tate, U.S., Moffet, B.S. and Hill, K. (1997) 'Reciprocity, emotional wellbeing and family functioning as determinants of family satisfaction in caregivers of elderly parents', *Nursing Research*, 46, 2, 93-100.

Charmaz, K. (2008) 'Views from the margins: Voices, silences, and suffering', *Qualitative Research in Psychology*, 5, 1, 7-18.

Chattoo, S. and Ahmad, W. (2008) 'The moral economy of selfhood and caring: Negotiating boundaries of personal care as embodied moral practice', *Sociology of Health & Illness*, 30, 4, 550-64.

Chen, J.H., Chan, D.C.D., Kiely, D.K., Morris, J.N. and Mitchell, S.L. (2007) 'Terminal trajectories of functional decline in the long-term care setting', *The Journals of Gerontology Series A: Biological Sciences and Medical Sciences*, 62, 5, 531-6.

Chenoweth, L., King, M.T., Jeon, Y.H., Brodaty, H., Stein-Parbury, J., Norman, R. et al (2009) 'Caring for Aged Dementia Care Resident Study (CADRES) of person-centred care, dementia-care mapping, and usual care in dementia: a cluster-randomised trial', *The Lancet Neurology*, 8, 4, 317-25.

Clare, L. (2010) 'Awareness in people with severe dementia: Review and integration', *Aging and Mental Health*, 14, 1, 20-32.

Clare, L., Markova, I., Verhey, F. and Kenny, G. (2005) 'Awareness in dementia: a review of assessment methods and measures', *Aging and Mental Health*, 9, 394-413.

Clarke, J.B. and Wheeler, S.J. (1992) 'A view of the phenomenon of caring in nursing practice', *Journal of Advanced Nursing*, 17, 11, 1283-90.

Clough, R. (1981) *Old age homes*, London: Allen & Unwin.

Cohen, D. and Eisdorfer, C. (2001) *The loss of self: A family resource for the care of Alzheimer's disease and related disorders*, New York, NY: WW Norton and Company.

Collard, R.M., Boter, H., Schoevers, R.A. and Oude Voshaar, R.C. (2012) 'Prevalence of frailty in community-dwelling older persons: a systematic review', *Journal of the American Geriatrics Society*, 60, 8, 1487-92.

Conlie Shaw, M.M. (1999) 'Nursing home resident abuse by staff: Exploring the dynamics', *Journal of Elder Abuse & Neglect*, 9, 4, 1-21.

Cook, K.S. (ed) (1987) *Social exchange theory*, Beverly Hills, CA: Sage Publications.

Cooley, C.H. (1922) *Human nature and the social order*, New York: C. Scribner & Sons.

Cornwell, J. (1984) *Hard earned lives: Accounts of health and illness from East London*, London: Tavistock.

Courtney, M., Tong, S. and Walsh, A. (2000) 'Acute-care nurses' attitudes towards older patients: A literature review', *International Journal of Nursing Practice*, 6, 62-9.

Covinsky, K.E., Eng, C., Lui, L.Y., Sands, L.P. and Yaffe, K. (2003) 'The last 2 years of life: functional trajectories of frail older people', *Journal of the American Geriatrics Society*, 51, 4, 492-8.

Crowther, M.A. (1982) *The workhouse system, 1834-1929*, Athens, GA: University of Georgia Press.

Cummins, R.A. (2001) 'The subjective well-being of people caring for a family member with a severe disability at home: A review', *Journal of Intellectual and Developmental Disability*, 26, 1, 83-100.

Curtis, B. (2002) 'Foucault on governmentality and population: The impossible discovery', *Canadian Journal of Sociology/Cahiers canadiens de sociologie*, 27, 4, 505-33.

Cutler, S.J. (2015) 'Worries about getting Alzheimer's: Who's concerned?', *American Journal of Alzheimer's Disease and Other Dementias* [online].

Dan-Cohen, M. (1992) 'Responsibility and the boundaries of the self', *Harvard Law Review*, 959-1003.

Davies, C. (2011) 'Preserving the "us identity" through marriage commitment while living with early-stage dementia', *Dementia*, 10, 2, 217-34.

Davies, N., Maio, L., Rait, G. and Iliffe, S. (2014) 'Quality end-of-life care for dementia: What have family carers told us so far? A narrative synthesis', *Palliative Medicine*, 28, 7, 919-30.

Dean, M. (1991) *The constitution of poverty: Towards a genealogy of liberal governance*, London: Routledge.

de Boer, M.E., Hertogh, C.M., Dröes, R.M., Jonker, C. and Eefsting, J.A. (2010) 'Advance directives in dementia: issues of validity and effectiveness', *International Psychogeriatrics*, 22, 2, 201-8.

de Boer, M.E., Hertogh, C.M., Dröes, R.M., Riphagen, I.I., Jonker, C. and Eefsting, J.A. (2007) 'Suffering from dementia – the patient's perspective: A review of the literature', *International Psychogeriatrics*, 19, 6, 1021-39.

de Ruijter, E. (2004) 'Trends in the outsourcing of domestic work and childcare in the Netherlands compositional or behavioral change?', *Acta Sociologica*, 47, 3, 219-34.

Degnen, C. (2007) 'Minding the gap: The construction of old age and oldness amongst peers', *Journal of Aging Studies*, 21, 1, 69-80.

Delp, L., Wallace, S.P., Geiger-Brown, J. and Muntaner, C. (2010) 'Job stress and job satisfaction: Home care workers in a consumer-directed model of care', *Health Services Research*, 45, 4, 922-40.

Del-Pino-Casado, R., Millán-Cobo, M.D., Palomino-Moral, P.A. and Frias-Osuna, A. (2014) 'Cultural correlates of burden in primary caregivers of older relatives: a cross-sectional study', *Journal of Nursing Scholarship*, 46, 3, 176-86.

Dennett, D. (1976) 'Conditions of personhood', in A.O. Rorty (ed) *The identities of persons*, Berkeley, CA: California University Press, pp 175-96.

Depp, C.A. and Jeste, D.V. (2006) 'Definitions and predictors of successful aging: a comprehensive review of larger quantitative studies', *The American Journal of Geriatric Psychiatry*, 14, 1, 6-20.

Dewey, R. (1948) 'Charles Horton Cooley: Pioneer in psychosociology', in H.E. Barnes (ed) *An introduction to the history of sociology*, Chicago, IL: University of Chicago Press, pp 833-52.

Dewing, J. (2008) 'Personhood and dementia: revisiting Tom Kitwood's ideas', *International Journal of Older People Nursing*, 3, 1, 3-13.

Dodson, L. and Zincavage, R.M. (2007) '"It's like a family": Caring labor, exploitation, and race in nursing homes', *Gender & Society*, 21, 6, 905-28.

Dowd, J.J. (1975) 'Aging as exchange: A preface to theory', *Journal of Gerontology*, 30, 5, 584-94.

Dowd, J.J. (1980) 'Exchange rates and old people', *Journal of Gerontology*, 35, 4, 596-602.

Downs, M. (1997) 'The emergence of the person in dementia research', *Ageing and Society*, 17, 5, 597-607.

Dresser, R. (1995) 'Dworkin on dementia: Elegant theory, questionable policy', *The Hastings Center Report*, 25, 6, 32-8.

Duffy, M. (2015) 'Beyond outsourcing: Paid care work in historical perspective', in M. Duffy, A. Armenia and C.L. Stacey (eds) *Caring on the clock: The complexities and contradictions of paid care work*, New Brunswick, NJ: Rutgers University Press, pp 14-26.

Duffy, M., Albelda, R. and Hammonds, C. (2013) 'Counting care work: The empirical and policy applications of care theory', *Social Problems*, 60, 2, 145-67.

Durkheim, E. (2005) 'The dualism of human nature and its social conditions', *Durkheimian Studies/Etudes durkheimiennes*, 11, 35-45.

Dworkin, R.M. (1993) *Life's dominion: An argument about abortion, euthanasia, and individual freedom*, New York: Alfred A. Knopf.

Dwyer, J.W., Lee, G.R. and Jankowski, T.B. (1994) 'Reciprocity, elder satisfaction and caregiver stress and burden: The exchange of aid in the family caregiving relationship', *Journal of Marriage and the Family*, 56, 35-43.

Dwyer, L.L., Nordenfelt, L. and Ternestedt, B.M. (2008) 'Three nursing home residents speak about meaning at the end of life', *Nursing Ethics*, 15, 1, 97-109.

Dyer, C. (2012) 'Poverty and its relief in late medieval England', *Past & Present*, 216, 1, 41-78.

Eastman, M. (1984) *Old age abuse*, Mitcham: Age Concern.

Eisdorfer, C., Cohen, D., Paveza, G.J. et al (1992) 'An empirical evaluation of the global deterioration scale for staging Alzheimer's disease', *American Journal of Psychiatry*, 149, 2, 190-4.

Elliott, C. (2001) *The self*, Cambridge: Polity Press.

Elofsson, L.C. and Öhlén, J. (2004) 'Meanings of being old and living with chronic obstructive pulmonary disease', *Palliative Medicine*, 18, 7, 611-18.

England, P. (2005) 'Emerging theories of care work', *Annual Review of Sociology*, 31, 381-99.

References

England, P., Folbre, N. and Leana, C. (2012) 'Motivating care', in N. Folbre (ed) *For love and money: Care provision in the United States*, New York: Russell Sage Foundation, pp 21-39.

Englander, D. (2013) *Poverty and Poor Law reform in nineteenth-century Britain, 1834-1914: From Chadwick to Booth*, London: Routledge.

Engster, D. (2005) 'Rethinking care theory: the practice of caring and the obligation to care', *Hypatia*, 20, 3, 50-74.

Esping-Andersen, G. (1999) *Social foundations of postindustrial economies*, Oxford: Oxford University Press.

Eustace, A., Coen, R., Walsh, C., Cunningham, C.J., Walsh, J.B., Coakley, D. and Lawlor, B.A. (2002) 'A longitudinal evaluation of behavioural and psychological symptoms of probable Alzheimer's disease', *International Journal of Geriatric Psychiatry*, 17, 10, 968-73.

Eymard, A.S. and Douglas D.H. (2012) 'Ageism among health care providers and interventions to improve their attitudes toward older adults: an integrative review', *Journal of Gerontological Nursing*, 38, 5, 26-35.

Farah, M.J. and Heberlein, A.S. (2007) 'Personhood and neuroscience: Naturalizing or nihilating?', *The American Journal of Bioethics*, 7, 1, 37-48.

Fazio, S. and Mitchell, D.B. (2009) 'Persistence of self in individuals with Alzheimer's disease: evidence from language and visual recognition', *Dementia*, 8, 39-59.

Finch, J. and Groves, D. (eds) (1983) *A labour of love: Women, work, and caring*, London: Routledge & Kegan Paul.

Fisher, A.L. (2005) 'Just what defines frailty?', *Journal of the American Geriatrics Society*, 53, 2229-30.

Fisher, B. and Tronto, J. (1990) 'Toward a feminist theory of caring', in E.K. Abel and M.K. Nelson (eds) *Circles of care: Work and identity in women's lives*, New York: State University of New York Press, pp 35-62.

Flatt, M.A., Settersten, R.A., Ponsaran, R. and Fishman, J.R. (2013) 'Are "anti-aging medicine" and "successful aging" two sides of the same coin? Views of anti-aging practitioners', *The Journals of Gerontology Series B: Psychological Sciences and Social Sciences*, 68, 6, 944-55.

Folbre, N. (ed) (2012) *For love and money: Care provision in the United States*, New York: Russell Sage Foundation.

Folbre, N. and Wright, E.O. (2012) 'Defining care', in N. Folbre (ed) *For love and money: Care provision in the United States*, New York: Russell Sage Foundation, pp 1-20.

Førsund, L.H., Skovdahl, K., Kiik, R. and Ytrehus, S. (2015) 'The loss of a shared lifetime: a qualitative study exploring spouses' experiences of losing couplehood with their partner with dementia living in institutional care', *Journal of Clinical Nursing*, 24, 1-2, 121-30.

Fortes, M. (1973) 'On the concept of the person among the Tallensi', in G. Dieterlen (ed) *La notion de la personne en Afrique Noire*, Paris: Éditions du Centre National de la Recherche Scientifique, pp 283-319.

Foucault, M. (2007) *Security, territory, population: Lectures at the Collège de France, 1977-1978* (translated by G. Burchell), New York: Palgrave Macmillan.

Frankfurt, H. (1971) 'Freedom of the will and the concept of a person', *The Journal of Philosophy*, 68, 1, 5-20.

Fraser, N. and Gordon, L. (1994) 'A genealogy of dependency: Tracing a keyword of the US welfare state', *Signs*, 19, 2, 309-36.

Fried, L.P. and Walston, J.M. (1998) 'Frailty and failure to thrive', in W.R. Hazzard, J.P. Blass, W.H. Ettinger et al (eds) *Principles of geriatric medicine and gerontology* (4th edn), New York: McGraw-Hill, pp 1487-502.

Fried, L.P., Ferrucci, L., Darer, J., Williamson, J.D. and Anderson, G. (2004) 'Untangling the concepts of disability, frailty and co-morbidity: Implications for improved targeting and care', *Journals of Gerontology: Medical Science*, 59A, 3, M255-63.

Fried, L.P., Tangen, C.M., Walston, J., Newman, A.B., Hirsch, C., Gottdiener, J. et al (2001) 'Frailty in older adults evidence for a phenotype', *Journals of Gerontology: Medical Science*, 56A, 3, M146-56.

Gallagher, S., Bennett, K.M. and Halford, J.C. (2006) 'A comparison of acute and long-term health-care personnel's attitudes towards older adults', *International Journal of Nursing Practice*, 12, 273-9.

Galvin, R. (2004) 'Challenging the need for gratitude comparisons between paid and unpaid care for disabled people', *Journal of Sociology*, 40, 2, 137-55.

Garcia-Garcia, F.J., Avila, G.G., Alfaro-Acha, A., Andres, M.A., Aparicio, M.E., Aparicio, S.H. and Rodríguez-Mañas, L. (2011) 'The prevalence of frailty syndrome in an older population from Spain. The Toledo Study for Healthy Aging', *The Journal of Nutrition, Health & Aging*, 15, 10, 852-6.

Gaugler, J.E., Zarit, S.H. and Pearlin, L.I. (2003) 'The onset of dementia caregiving and its longitudinal implications', *Psychology and Aging*, 18, 2, 171-80.

Geertz, C. (1994) 'Thick description: Toward an interpretive theory of culture', *Readings in the Philosophy of Social Science*, 213-31.

References

Gellis, Z.D., Sherman, S. and Lawrance, F. (2003) 'First year graduate social work students' knowledge of and attitude toward older adults', *Educational Gerontology*, 29, 1, 1-16.

Geremek, B. (1997) *Poverty: A history*, Oxford: Blackwell.

Gerstorf, D. and Ram, N. (2013) 'Inquiry into terminal decline: five objectives for future study', *The Gerontologist*, 53, 5, 727-37.

Gerstorf, D., Ram, N., Lindenberger, U. and Smith, J. (2013) 'Age and time-to-death trajectories of change in indicators of cognitive, sensory, physical, health, social, and self-related functions', *Developmental Psychology*, 49, 10, 1805-11.

Gerstorf, D., Ram, N., Mayraz, G., Hidajat, M., Lindenberger, U., Wagner, G.G. and Schupp, J. (2010) 'Late-life decline in well-being across adulthood in Germany, the United Kingdom, and the United States: Something is seriously wrong at the end of life', *Psychology and Aging*, 25, 2, 477-85.

Giddens, A. (1984) *The constitution of society*, Cambridge: Polity Press.

Giddens, A. (1990) *The consequences of modernity*, Cambridge: Polity Press.

Giddens, A. (1991) *Modernity and self-identity. Self and society in the late modern age*, Cambridge: Polity Press.

Gilleard, C.J. and Higgs, P. (1998) 'Old people as users and consumers of healthcare: a third age rhetoric for a fourth age reality?', *Ageing and Society*, 18, 2, 233-48.

Gilleard, C.J. and Higgs, P. (2000) *Cultures of ageing: Self, citizen, and the body*, Harlow: Pearson Education.

Gilleard, C.J. and Higgs, P. (2005) *Contexts of ageing: Class, cohort and community*, Cambridge: Polity Press.

Gilleard, C.J. and Higgs, P. (2010) 'Aging without agency: Theorizing the fourth age', *Aging & Mental Health*, 14, 2, 121-8.

Gilleard, C.J. and Higgs, P. (2011a) 'Frailty, disability and old age: A re-appraisal', *Health*, 15, 5, 475-90.

Gilleard, C.J. and Higgs, P. (2011b) 'Aging, abjection and embodiment in the fourth age', *Journal of Aging Studies*, 25, 2, 135-42.

Gilleard, C.J. and Higgs, P. (2013) 'The fourth age and the concept of a "social imaginary": A theoretical excursus', *Journal of Aging Studies*, 27, 4, 368-76.

Gilleard, C.J. and Higgs, P. (2015) 'Social death and the moral identity of the fourth age', *Contemporary Social Science*, 10, 3, 262-71.

Gilleard, C.J. and Higgs, P. (2016) 'Ageing corporeality and the social divisions of later life', *Ageing & Society* [in press].

Gillies, B. (2012) 'Continuity and loss: The carer's journey through dementia', *Dementia*, 11, 5, 657-76.

Gilligan, C. (1982) *In a different voice*, Cambridge, MA: Harvard University Press.

Gobbens, R.J., van Assen, M.A., Luijkx, K.G., Wijnen-Sponselee, M.T. and Schols, J.M. (2010) 'Determinants of frailty', *Journal of the American Medical Directors Association*, 11, 5, 356-64.

Goffman, E. (1961) *Asylums*, Harmondsworth: Penguin Books.

Goffman, E. (1959/1971) *The presentation of self in everyday life*, Harmondsworth: Penguin Books.

Goffman, E. (1990) *Stigma: Notes on the management of spoiled identity*, Harmondsworth: Penguin Books.

Goldman, L. (1991) 'Statistics and the science of society in early Victorian Britain: An intellectual context for the General Register Office', *Social History of Medicine*, 4, 3, 415-34.

Goodman, C., Evans, C., Wilcock, J., Froggatt, K., Drennan, V., Sampson, E. et al (2010) 'End of life care for community dwelling older people with dementia: an integrated review', *International Journal of Geriatric Psychiatry*, 25, 4, 329-37.

Goodridge, D.M., Johnston, P. and Thomson, M. (1996) 'Conflict and aggression as stressors in the work environment of nursing assistants: Implications for institutional elder abuse', *Journal of Elder Abuse & Neglect*, 8, 1, 49-67.

Gordijn, B. (1999) 'The troublesome concept of the person', *Theoretical Medicine and Bioethics*, 20, 4, 347-59.

Gouldner, A.W. (1973) 'The norm of reciprocity: a preliminary statement' in A.W. Gouldner (ed), *For sociology*, London: Allan Lane, pp 226-59.

Graham, J.E. and Bassett, R. (2006) 'Reciprocal relations: The recognition and co-construction of caring with Alzheimer's disease', *Journal of Aging Studies*, 20, 4, 335-49.

Grau, L., Chandler, B. and Saunders, C. (1995) 'Nursing home residents' perceptions of the quality of their care', *Journal of Psychosocial Nursing & Mental Health Services*, 33, 5, 34-41.

Green, M. and Lawson, V. (2011) 'Recentring care: interrogating the commodification of care', *Social & Cultural Geography*, 12, 6, 639-54.

Gregson, N., Crang, M., Botticello, J., Calestani, M. and Krzywoszynska, A. (2014) 'Doing the "dirty work" of the green economy: Resource recovery and migrant labour in the EU', *European Urban and Regional Studies*, doi: 0969776414554489.

Grenier, A. (2007) 'Constructions of frailty in the English language, care practice and the lived experience', *Ageing & Society*, 27, 3, 425-46.

Grenier, A. and Hanley, J. (2007) 'Older women and "frailty": Aged, gendered and embodied resistance', *Current Sociology*, 55, 2, 211-28.

Griffin, D.R. (2013) *Animal minds: Beyond cognition to consciousness*, Chicago, IL: University of Chicago Press.

Grill, J.D., Zhou, Y., Karlawish, J. and Elashoff, D. (2014) 'Does study partner type impact the rate of Alzheimer's disease progression?', *Journal of Alzheimer's Disease*, 38, 3, 507-14.

Grov, E.K. and Valeberg, B.T. (2012) 'Does the cancer patient's disease stage matter? A comparative study of caregivers' mental health and health related quality of life', *Palliative and Supportive Care*, 10, 2, 189-96.

Hall, E.O. and Høy, B. (2012) 'Re-establishing dignity: nurses' experiences of caring for older hospital patients', *Scandinavian Journal of Caring Sciences*, 26, 2, 287-94.

Hall, S., Longhurst, S. and Higginson, I. (2009) 'Living and dying with dignity: a qualitative study of the views of older people in nursing homes', *Age and Ageing*, 38, 4, 411-16.

Halwani, R. (2003) 'Care ethics and virtue ethics', *Hypatia*, 18, 3, 161-92.

Harrefors, C., Sävenstedt, S. and Axelsson, K. (2009) 'Elderly people's perceptions of how they want to be cared for: an interview study with healthy elderly couples in Northern Sweden', *Scandinavian Journal of Caring Sciences*, 23, 2, 353-60.

Harris, P.B. (2002) *The person with Alzheimer's disease: Pathways to understanding the experience*, Baltimore, MD: Johns Hopkins University Press.

Harrison, J.K., Clegg, A., Conroy, S.P. and Young, J. (2015) 'Managing frailty as a long-term condition', *Age and Ageing*, 44, 5, 733-35.

Hart, E.A. (1866) *An account of the condition of the infirmaries of London workhouses*, London: Chapman & Hall.

Hedinger, D., Braun, J., Zellweger, U., Kaplan, V., Bopp M. et al (2014) 'Moving to and dying in a nursing home depends not only on health – An analysis of socio-demographic determinants of place of death in Switzerland', *PLoS ONE*, 9, 11, e113236.

Hegel, G.W.F. (1991) *Elements of the philosophy of right* (translated by H.B. Nisbet, edited by A.W. Wood), Cambridge: Cambridge University Press.

Held, T. (1986) 'Institutionalization and deinstitutionalization of the life course', *Human Development*, 29, 3, 157-62.

Hellstrom, I., Nolan, M. and Lundh, U. (2007) 'Sustaining "couplehood": spouses' strategies for living positively with dementia', *Dementia*, 6, 383-409.

Hennings, J., Froggatt, K. and Payne, S. (2013) 'Spouse caregivers of people with advanced dementia in nursing homes: A longitudinal narrative study', *Palliative Medicine*, 27, 7, 683-91.

Henson, R.H. (1997) 'Analysis of the concept of mutuality', *Image: the Journal of Nursing Scholarship*, 29, 1, 77-81.

Hertogh, C.M. (2011) 'The misleading simplicity of advance directives', *International Psychogeriatrics*, 23, 4, 511-15.

Heru, A.M. and Ryan, C.E. (2006) 'Family functioning in the caregivers of patients with dementia: One-year follow-up', *Bulletin of the Menninger Clinic*, 70, 3, 222-31.

Higgs, E. (2004) *The information state in England: The central collection of information on citizens since 1500*, London: Palgrave Macmillan.

Higgs, P. (2012) 'Consuming bodies: Zygmunt Bauman on the difference between fitness and health', in G. Scambler (ed) *Contemporary theorists for medical sociology*, London: Routledge, pp 20-32.

Higgs, P. and Gilleard, C.J. (2014) 'Frailty, abjection and the "othering" of the fourth age', *Health Sociology Review*, 23, 1, 10-19.

Higgs, P. and Gilleard, C.J. (2015) *Rethinking old age: Theorising the fourth age*, London: Palgrave Macmillan.

Higgs, P. and Gilleard, C.J. (2016) 'Interrogating personhood and dementia', *Aging & Mental Health*, 20, 8, 773-80.

Himmelfarb, G. (1984) *The idea of poverty: England in the early Industrial Age*, New York: Knopf.

Himmelfarb, G. (1991) *Poverty and compassion: The moral imagination of the late Victorians*, New York: Knopf.

Himmelweit, S. (1999) 'Caring labor', *The Annals of the American Academy of Political and Social Science*, 561, 1, 27-38.

Hirsch, C., Anderson, M.L., Newman, A., Kop, W., Jackson, S., Gottdiener, J., Tracy, R., Fried, L. and Cardiovascular Health Study Research Group (2006) 'The association of race with frailty: the cardiovascular health study', *Annals of Epidemiology*, 16, 7, 545-53.

Hirschfeld, M. (1983) 'Home care versus institutionalization: family caregiving and senile brain disease', *International Journal of Nursing Studies*, 20, 1, 23-32.

Hirschman, K.B., Kapo, J.M. and Karlawish, J.H.T. (2006) 'Why doesn't a family member of a person with advanced dementia use a substituted judgment when making a decision for that person?', *American Journal of Geriatric Psychiatry*, 14, 8, 659-67.

Hirshbein, L.D. (2000) '"Normal" old age, senility, and the American Geriatrics Society in the 1940s', *Journal of the History of Medicine and Allied Sciences*, 55, 4, 337-62.

References

Hochschild, A.R. (1997) *The time bind: When work becomes home and home becomes work*, New York: Metropolitan Books.

Hochschild, A.R. (2003) *The managed heart: Commercialization of human feeling*, Berkeley, CA: University of California Press.

Hodgkiss, P. (2001) *The making of the modern mind: The surfacing of consciousness in social thought*, London: Athlone Press.

Hogan, D.B., Freiheit, E.A., Strain, L.A., Patten, S.B., Schmaltz, H.N., Rolfson, D. and Maxwell, C.J. (2012) 'Comparing frailty measures in their ability to predict adverse outcome among older residents of assisted living', *BMC Geriatrics*, 12, 1, 56, 1-11.

Hondagneu-Sotelo, P. (2001) *Domestica: Immigrant workers cleaning and caring in the shadows of affluence*, Berkeley, CA: University of California Press.

Hope, R.A., Keane, J., Fairburn, C., McShane, R. and Jacoby, R. (1997) 'Behaviour changes in dementia II: Are there behavioural syndromes?', *International Journal of Geriatric Psychiatry*, 12, 1074-78.

Horowitz, A. and Shindelman, L.W. (1983) 'Reciprocity and affection: Past influences on current caregiving', *Journal of Gerontological Social Work*, 5, 3, 5-20.

Houttekier, D., Cohen, J., Surkyn, J. and Deliens, L. (2011) 'Study of recent and future trends in place of death in Belgium using death certificate data: a shift from hospitals to care homes', *BMC Public Health*, 11, 1, 228.

Houttekier, D., Cohen, J., Bilsen, J., Addington-Hall, J., Onwuteaka-Philipsen, B.D. and Deliens, L. (2010) 'Place of death of older persons with dementia. A study in five European countries', *Journal of the American Geriatrics Society*, 58, 4, 751-6.

Howes, C. (2005) 'Living waged and retention of homecare workers in San Francisco', *Industrial Relations*, 44, 1, 139-63.

Howes, C. (2008) 'Love, money, or flexibility: what motivates people to work in consumer-directed home care?', *The Gerontologist*, 48, Special Issue I, 46-59.

Howorth, P. and Saper, J. (2003) 'The dimensions of insight in people with dementia'. *Aging and Mental Health*, 7, 113-22.

Hrdy, S.B. (1999) *Mother nature: A history of mothers, infants and natural selection*, New York: Pantheon Books.

Hubbard, G. and Forbat, L. (2012) 'Cancer as biographical disruption: constructions of living with cancer', *Supportive Care in Cancer*, 20, 9, 2033-40.

Hubbard, G., Downs, M.G. and Tester, S. (2003) 'Including older people with dementia in research: Challenges and strategies', *Aging & Mental Health*, 7, 5, 351-62.

Hughes, B., McKie, L., Hopkins, D. and Watson, N. (2005) 'Love's labours lost? Feminism, the disabled people's movement and an ethic of care', *Sociology*, 39, 2, 259-75.

Hughes, C.P., Berg, L., Danziger, W.L., Coben, L.A. and Martin, R.L. (1982) 'A new clinical scale for the staging of dementia', *The British Journal of Psychiatry*, 140, 6, 566-72.

Hughes, J.C. (2013) 'Philosophical issues in dementia', *Current Opinion in Psychiatry*, 26, 3, 283-8.

Hughes, J.C., Louw, S.J. and Sabat, S.R. (eds) (2006) *Dementia: Mind, meaning, and the person*, Oxford: Oxford University Press.

Hume, D. (1978) *A treatise of human nature* (2nd edn) (edited and revised by P.H. Nidditch), Oxford: Clarendon Press.

Hung, W.W., Ross, J.S., Boockvar, K.S. and Siu, A.L. (2012) 'Association of chronic diseases and impairments with disability in older adults: a decade of change?', *Medical Care*, 50, 6, 501.

Hussein, S. and Manthorpe, J. (2014) 'Structural marginalisation among the long-term care workforce in England: evidence from mixed-effect models of national pay data', *Ageing & Society*, 34, 1, 21-41.

Hussein, S., Ismail, M. and Manthorpe, J. (2015) 'Changes in turnover and vacancy rates of care workers in England from 2008 to 2010: panel analysis of national workforce data', *Health and Social Care in the Community*, doi: 10.1111/hsc.12214.

Hutchison, A. and Stenfert Kroese, B. (2015) 'A review of literature exploring the possible causes of abuse and neglect in adult residential care', *The Journal of Adult Protection*, 17, 4, 216-33.

Hyde, M. and Higgs, P. (2016) *Ageing and globalisation*, Bristol: Policy Press.

Iecovich, E. (2011) 'What makes migrant live-in home care workers in elder care be satisfied with their job?', *The Gerontologist*, 51, 5, 617-29.

Innes, A., Archibald, C. and Murphy, C. (2004) *Dementia and social inclusion: Marginalised groups and marginalised areas of dementia research, care and practice*, London: Jessica Kingsley Publishers.

Isaksson, U., Graneheim, U.H. and Åström, S. (2009) 'Female caregivers' experiences of exposure to violence in nursing homes', *Journal of Psychiatric and Mental Health Nursing*, 16, 1, 46-53.

James, N. (1992) 'Care = organisation + physical labour + emotional labour', *Sociology of Health and Illness*, 14, 4, 488-509.

Jaworska, A. (1999) 'Respecting the margins of agency: Alzheimer's patients and the capacity to value', *Philosophy & Public Affairs*, 28, 2, 105-38.

Jenkins, D. and Price, B. (1996) 'Dementia and personhood: A focus for care?', *Journal of Advanced Nursing*, 24, 84-90.

Jenkins, R. (1997) *Social identity*, London: Routledge.

Jenkins, S.P. (2015) *The income distribution in the UK: A picture of advantage and disadvantage*, IZA Discussion Papers, No 8835, Bonn: Institute for the Study of Labor (IZA) (http://hdl.handle.net/10419/108716).

Jetten, J., Haslam, C., Pugliese, C., Tonks, J. and Haslam, S.A. (2010) 'Declining autobiographical memory and the loss of identity: Effects on well-being', *Journal of Clinical and Experimental Neuropsychology*, 32, 4, 408-16.

Johnson, M.L. (1995) 'Interdependency and the generational compact', *Ageing & Society*, 15, 2, 243-65.

Jütte, R. (1994) *Poverty and deviance in early modern Europe*, Cambridge: Cambridge University Press.

Kahn, R.L. (2002) 'Guest editorial: on "Successful aging and well-being: self-rated compared with Rowe and Kahn"', *The Gerontologist*, 42, 6, 725-26.

Kant, I. (1895) *Fundamental principles of the metaphysics of ethics* (translated by T. Kingsmill Abbott), London: Longmans, Green & Co.

Kaufman, S. (1994) 'The social construction of frailty: An anthropological perspective', *Journal of Aging Studies*, 8, 1, 45-58.

Kelaiditi, E., Cesari, M., Canevelli, M., van Kan, G.A., Ousset, P.J., Gillette-Guyonnet, S., Ritz, P. and Vellas, B. (2013) 'Cognitive frailty: rational and definition from an (IANA/IAGG) international consensus group', *The Journal of Nutrition, Health & Aging*, 17, 9, 726-34.

Kittay, E.F. (1999) *Love's labor: Essays on women, equality, dependency*, New York: Routledge.

Kittay, E.F. and Carlson, L. (eds) (2010) *Cognitive disability and its challenge to moral philosophy*, London: Wiley-Blackwell.

Kitwood, T.M. (1993) 'Towards a theory of dementia care: the interpersonal process', *Ageing & Society*, 13, 1, 51-67.

Kitwood, T.M. (1997a) *Dementia reconsidered. The person comes first*, Buckingham: Open University Press.

Kitwood, T.M. (1997b) 'The concept of personhood and its relevance for a new culture of dementia care', in B.M.L. Meisen and G.M.M. Jones (eds) *Care-giving in dementia, research and applications*, vol 2, London, Routledge, pp 3-13.

Kitwood, T.M. and Benson, S. (eds) (1995) *The new culture of dementia care*, London: Hawker.

Kitwood, T.M. and Bredin, K. (1992) 'Towards a theory of dementia care: personhood and well-being', *Ageing & Society*, 12, 3, 269-87.

Kleemeier, R.W. (1962) 'Intellectual changes in the senium', *Proceedings of the American Statistical Association*, 1, 290-5.

Korsgaard, C.M. (1989) 'Personal identity and the unity of agency: A Kantian response to Parfit', *Philosophy & Public Affairs*, 18, 2, 101-32.

Kristeva, J. (1982) *Powers of horror: An essay on abjection*, New York: Columbia University Press.

Kulmala, J., Nykänen, I., Mänty, M. and Hartikainen, S. (2014) 'Association between frailty and dementia: A population-based study', *Gerontology*, 60, 1, 16-21.

Lachs, M.S., Rosen, T., Teresi, J.A., Eimicke, J.P., Ramirez, M., Silver, S. and Pillemer, K. (2013) 'Verbal and physical aggression directed at nursing home staff by residents', *Journal of General Internal Medicine*, 28, 5, 660-7.

Laslett, B. and Brenner, J. (1989) 'Gender and social reproduction: Historical perspectives', *Annual Review of Sociology*, 15, 381-404.

Laslett, P. (1989) *A fresh map of life*, London: Weidenfeld & Nicolson.

Laslett, P. (1996) *A fresh map of life, 2nd ed*, London: Macmillan.

Lawrehce, V., Fossey, J., Ballard, C., Moniz-Cook, E. and Murray, J. (2012) 'Improving quality of life for people with dementia in care homes: making psychosocial interventions work', *British Journal of Psychiatry*, 201, 5, 344-51.

Lawson, H. (1985) *Reflexivity: The post-modern predicament*, London: Hutchinson.

Leaf, A. (1982) 'Long-lived populations: Extreme old age', *Journal of the American Geriatrics Society*, 30, 485-7.

Lee, R.P., Bamford, C., Exley, C. and Robinson, L. (2015) 'Expert views on the factors enabling good end of life care for people with dementia: a qualitative study', *BMC Palliative Care*, 14, 1, 32.

Lee-Treweek, G. (1997) 'Women, resistance and care: An ethnographic study of nursing auxiliary work', *Work, Employment & Society*, 11, 1, 47-63.

Leira, A. (1994) 'Concepts of caring: Loving, thinking, and doing', *The Social Service Review*, 68, 2, 185-201.

Lewinter, M. (2003) 'Reciprocities in caregiving relationships in Danish elder care', *Journal of Aging Studies*, 17, 3, 357-77.

Llewellyn, H., Low, J., Smith, G., Hopkins, K., Burns, A. and Jones, L. (2014) 'Narratives of continuity among older people with late stage chronic kidney disease who decline dialysis', *Social Science & Medicine*, 114, 49-56.

Locke, J. (1975) *An essay concerning human understanding* (edited by P.H. Nidditch), Oxford: Clarendon Press.

London, J. (1903) *The people of the abyss*, London: Macmillan.

Longmate, N. (2003) *The workhouse: A social history*, London: Random House.

References

Lopez, S.H. (2006) 'Emotional labor and organized emotional care conceptualizing nursing home care work', *Work and Occupations*, 33, 2, 133-60.

Low, J., Myers, J., Smith, G., Higgs, P., Burns, A., Hopkins, K. and Jones, L. (2014) 'The experiences of close persons caring for people with chronic kidney disease stage 5 on conservative kidney management: Contested discourses of ageing', *Health*, 18, 6, 613-30.

Luppa, M., Luck, T., Brähler, E., König, H.H. and Riedel-Heller, S.G. (2008) 'Prediction of institutionalisation in dementia', *Dementia and Geriatric Cognitive Disorders*, 26, 1, 65-78.

Luppa, M., Luck, T., Matschinger, H., König, H.H. and Riedel-Heller, S.G. (2010a) 'Predictors of nursing home admission of individuals without a dementia diagnosis before admission-results from the Leipzig Longitudinal Study of the Aged (LEILA 75+)', *BMC Health Services Research*, 10, 1, 186.

Luppa, M., Luck, T., Weyerer, S., König, H.-H., Brähler, E. and Riedel-Heller, S.G. (2010b) 'Prediction of institutionalization in the elderly: A systematic review', *Age and Ageing*, 39, 1, 31-8.

Lyotard, J.F. (1984) *The postmodern condition: A report on knowledge*, Minneapolis, MN: University of Minnesota Press.

McCarthy, M., Addington-Hall, J. and Altmann, D. (1997) 'The experience of dying with dementia: a retrospective study', *International Journal of Geriatric Psychiatry*, 12, 4, 404-9.

McCormack, B. (2001) *Negotiating partnerships with older people: A person centred approach*, Aldershot: Ashgate Publishing.

McCormack, B. (2004) 'Person-centredness in gerontological nursing: an overview of the literature', *Journal of Clinical Nursing*, 13, 3a, 31-8.

McDonald, L., Beaulieu, M., Harbison, J., Hirst, S., Lowenstein, A., Podnieks, E. and Wahl, J. (2012) 'Institutional abuse of older adults: What we know, what we need to know', *Journal of Elder Abuse & Neglect*, 24, 2, 138-60.

McKee, K., Downs, M., Gilhooly, M., Gilhooly, K., Tester, S. and Wilson, F. (2005) 'Frailty, identity and the quality of later life', in A. Walker (ed) *Understanding quality of life in old age*, London: McGraw-Hill Education, pp 117-29.

McLafferty, I. and Morrison, F. (2004) 'Attitudes toward hospitalized older adults', *Journal of Advanced Nursing*, 47, 4, 446-53.

Majer, I.M., Nusselder, W.J., Mackenbach, J.P. and Kunst, A.E. (2011) 'Socioeconomic inequalities in life and health expectancies around official retirement age in 10 Western-European countries', *Journal of Epidemiology and Community Health*, 65, 11, 972-9.

Malmedal, W., Hammervold, R. and Saveman, B.I. (2014) 'The dark side of Norwegian nursing homes: factors influencing inadequate care', *The Journal of Adult Protection*, 16, 3, 133-51.

Manthorpe, J. (2015) 'Elder abuse', in I.B. Crome, L.-T. Wu, R. Rao and P. Crome (eds) *Substance use and older people*, Chichester: John Wiley & Sons, pp 11-17.

Marshall, T.H. (1992) *Citizenship and social class*, London: Pluto Press.

Martikainen, P., Moustgaard, H., Murphy, M., Einiö, E.K., Koskinen, S., Martelin, T. and Noro, A. (2009) 'Gender, living arrangements, and social circumstances as determinants of entry into and exit from long-term institutional care at older ages: A 6-year follow-up study of older Finns', *The Gerontologist*, 49, 1, 34-45.

Marx, K. (2002) 'The *Eighteenth Brumaire* of Louis Bonaparte', in M. Cowling and J. Martin (eds) *Marx's 'Eighteenth Brumaire': (Post)modern interpretations*, London: Pluto Press, pp 19-109.

Mathieson, C.M. and Stam, H.J. (1995) 'Renegotiating identity: cancer narratives', *Sociology of Health & Illness*, 17, 3, 283-306.

Mauss, M. (1938/1985) 'A category of the human mind: the notion of person, the notion of self', in M. Carrithers, S. Collins and S. Lukes (eds) *The category of the person: Anthropology, philosophy, history*, Cambridge: Cambridge University Press, pp 1-25.

McGovern, J. (2011) 'Couple meaning-making and dementia: challenges to the deficit model', *Journal of Gerontological Social Work*, 54, 678-90.

McLaughlin, T., Feldman, H., Fillit, H., Sano, M., Schmitt, F., Aisen, P., Leibman, C., Mucha, L., Ryan, J.M., Sullivan, S.D. and Spackman, D.E. (2010) 'Dependence as a unifying construct in defining Alzheimer's disease severity', *Alzheimer's and Dementia*, 6, 6, 482-93.

Meacher, M. (1972) *Taken for a ride: Special residential homes for confused old people: A study of separatism in social policy*, London: Longman.

Mead, G.H. (1935/1962) *Mind, self and society* (edited by C.W. Morris), Chicago, IL: University of Chicago Press.

Meagher, G. (2006) 'What can we expect from paid carers?', *Politics & Society*, 34, 1, 33-54.

Meiboom, A.A., de Vries, H., Hertogh, C.M. and Scheele, F. (2015) 'Why medical students do not choose a career in geriatrics: a systematic review', *BMC Medical Education*, 15, 1, 101.

Middleton, J. (1973) 'The concept of the person among the Lugbara of Uganda', in G. Dieterlen (ed) *La notion de personne en Afrique Noire*, Paris: Editions du Centre National de la Recherche Scientifique, pp 491-506.

Miller, S.C., Lepore, M., Lima, J.C., Shield, R. and Tyler, D.A. (2014) 'Does the introduction of nursing home culture change practices improve quality?', *Journal of the American Geriatrics Society*, 62, 9, 1675-82.

Mischel, W. (1974) 'Processes in delay of gratification', in L. Berkowitz (ed) *Advances in experimental social psychology*, vol 7, New York: Academic Press, pp 249-92.

Mitchell, S.L., Teno, J.M., Miller, S.C. et al (2005) 'A national study of the location of death for older persons with dementia', *Journal of the American Geriatrics Society*, 53, 2, 299-305.

Mitchell, S.L., Teno, J.M., Kiely, D.K., Shaffer, M.L., Jones, R.N., Prigerson, H.G. et al (2009) 'The clinical course of advanced dementia', *New England Journal of Medicine*, 361, 16, 1529-38.

Mitnitski, A.B., Graham, J.E., Mogilner, A.J. and Rockwood, K. (2002a) 'Frailty, fitness and late-life mortality in relation to chronological and biological age', *BMC Geriatrics*, 2, 1, 1.

Mitnitski, A.B., Mogilner, A.J., MacKnight, C. and Rockwood, K. (2002b) 'The mortality rate as a function of accumulated deficits in a frailty index', *Mechanisms of Ageing and Development*, 123, 11, 1457-60.

Mollat, M. (1986) *The poor in the Middle Ages: An essay in social history* (translated by A. Goldhammer), New Haven, CT: Yale University Press.

Montgomery, R.J.V., Lyn, H., Deichert, J. and Kosloski, K. (2005) 'A profile of home care workers from the 2000 census: how it changes what we know', *The Gerontologist*, 45, 5, 595-600.

Mooney, M.A. (2014) 'Virtues and human personhood in the social sciences', in V. Jeffries (ed) *The Palgrave Handbook of Altruism, Morality, and Social Solidarity*, London: Palgrave Macmillan, pp 21-41.

Morgan, D.G., Cammer, A., Stewart, N.J., Crossley, M., D'Arcy, C., Forbes, D.A. and Karunanayake, C. (2012) 'Nursing aide reports of combative behavior by residents with dementia: results from a detailed prospective incident diary', *Journal of the American Medical Directors Association*, 13, 3, 220-7.

Morris, J. (2001) 'Impairment and disability: constructing an ethics of care that promotes human rights', *Hypatia*, 16, 4, 1-16.

Morris, L.W., Morris, R.G. and Britton, P.G. (1988) 'The relationship between marital intimacy, perceived strain and depression in spouse caregivers of dementia sufferers', *British Journal of Medical Psychology*, 61, 3, 231-6.

Mulkay, M. (1992) 'Social death in Britain', *The Sociological Review*, 40, S1 31-49.

Munnichs, J.M.A. (1976) 'Dependency, interdependency and autonomy: An introduction', in J.M.A. Munnichs and W.J.A. van den Heuvel (eds) *Dependency or interdependency in old age*, Dordrecht: Springer, pp 3-8.

Nakrem, S., Vinsnes, A.G. and Seim, A. (2011) 'Residents' experiences of interpersonal factors in nursing home care: a qualitative study', *International Journal of Nursing Studies*, 48, 11, 1357-66.

Nakrem, S., Vinsnes, A.G., Harkless, G.E., Paulsen, B. and Seim, A. (2013) 'Ambiguities: residents' experience of "nursing home as my home"', *International Journal of Older People Nursing*, 8, 3, 216-25.

Nelson, J.A. (1999) 'Of markets and martyrs: Is it OK to pay well for care?', *Feminist Economics*, 5, 3, 43-59.

Neugarten, B.L. (1974) 'Age groups in American society and the rise of the young-old', *The Annals of the American Academy of Political and Social Science*, 415, 1, 187-98.

NICE (2006) *Dementia: supporting people with dementia and their carers in health and social care*, London: National Institute for Health and Care Excellence.

Nicholson, C., Meyer, J., Flatley, M., Holman, C. and Lowton, K. (2012) 'Living on the margin: understanding the experience of living and dying with frailty in old age', *Social Science & Medicine*, 75, 8, 1426-32.

Nietzsche, F. (1994) *On the genealogy of morality*, Cambridge: Cambridge University Press.

Noddings, N. (1984) *Caring: A feminine approach to ethics and moral education*, Berkeley, CA: University of California Press.

Norton, M.C., Piercy, K.W., Rabins, P.V., Green, R.C., Breitner, J.C., Østbye, T. et al (2009) 'Caregiver–recipient closeness and symptom progression in Alzheimer disease. The Cache county dementia progression study', *The Journals of Gerontology Series B: Psychological Sciences and Social Sciences*, 64, 5, 560-8.

Nuffield Council on Bioethics (2009) *Dementia: ethical issues*, London: Nuffield Council on Bioethics.

Nussbaum, M. (2000) *Women and human development: The capabilities approach*, Cambridge: Cambridge University Press.

O'Connor, D.L. (2007) 'Self-identifying as a caregiver: Exploring the positioning process', *Journal of Aging Studies*, 21, 3, 163-74.

Ohlén, J., Ekman, I., Zingmark, K., Bolmsjö, I. and Benzein, E. (2014) 'Conceptual development of "at-homeness" despite illness and disease: a review', *International Journal of Qualitative Studies on Health and Well-Being*, 9, 23677.

Ohlin, J.D. (2005) 'Is the concept of the person necessary for human rights?', *Columbia Law Review*, 105, 1, 209-49.

Okin, S.M., (2003/4) Justice and Gender: An Unfinished Debate. *Fordham Law Review*, 72, 1537-1567.

Oliver, M. (1989) 'Disability and dependency: A creation of industrial societies?', in L. Barton (ed) *Disability and dependency*, Lewes: Falmer Press, pp 7-22.

Oropesa, R.S. (1993) 'Using the service economy to relieve the double burden: Female labor force participation and service purchases', *Journal of Family Issues*, 14, 438-73.

Outhwaite, W. (2009) 'Canon formation in late 20th-century British sociology', *Sociology*, 43, 6, 1029-45.

Page, S. and Keady, J. (2010) 'Sharing stories : a meta-ethnographic analysis of 12 autobiographies written by people with dementia between 1989 and 2007', *Ageing & Society*, 30, 5, 511-26.

Paley, J. (2002) 'Caring as a slave morality: Nietzschean themes in nursing ethics', *Journal of Advanced Nursing*, 40, 1, 25-35.

Palmer, E. and Eveline, J. (2012) 'Sustaining low pay in aged care work', *Gender, Work & Organization*, 19, 3, 254-75.

Palmer, J.A., Meterko, M., Zhao, S., Berlowitz, D., Mobley, E. and Hartmann, C.W. (2013) 'Nursing home employee perceptions of culture change', *Research in Gerontological Nursing*, 6, 3, 152.

Palmore, E. and Cleveland, W. (1976) 'Aging, terminal decline, and terminal drop', *Journal of Gerontology*, 31, 1, 76-81.

Panza, F., d'Introno, A., Colacicco, A.M., Capurso, C., Del Parigi, A., Capurso, S.A., Caselli, R.J. and Solfrizzi, V. (2006) 'Cognitive frailty: predementia syndrome and vascular risk factors', *Neurobiology of Aging*, 27, 7, 933-40.

Parfit, D. (1984) *Reasons and persons*, Oxford: Oxford University Press.

Parfit, D. (2003a) 'Why our identity is not what matters', in R. Martin and J. Barresi (eds) *Personal identity*, Oxford: Blackwell, pp 115-43.

Parfit, D. (2003b) 'The unimportance of identity', in R. Martin and J. Barresi (eds) *Personal identity*, Oxford: Blackwell, pp 292-317.

Parker, G. (1990) *With due care and attention: A review of research on informal care* (2nd edn), London: Family Policy Studies Centre.

Parton, N. (2003) 'Rethinking professional practice: The contributions of social constructionism and the feminist "ethics of care"', *British Journal of Social Work*, 33, 1, 1-16.

Perring, C. (1997) 'Degrees of personhood', *The Journal of Medicine and Philosophy*, 2, 173-97.

Perry, E.K. (1986) 'The cholinergic hypothesis – ten years on', *British Medical Bulletin*, 42, 1, 63-9.

Piaget, J. (1976) *The grasp of consciousness: Action and concept in the young child*, Cambridge, MA: Harvard University Press.

Pinnock, H., Kendall, M., Murray, S.A., Worth, A., Levack, P., Porter, M. et al (2011) 'Living and dying with severe chronic obstructive pulmonary disease: multi-perspective longitudinal qualitative study', *BMJ*, 342, d142.

Pinquart, M. and Sörensen, S. (2003) 'Associations of stressors and uplifts of caregiving with caregiver burden and depressive mood: a meta-analysis', *The Journals of Gerontology Series B: Psychological Sciences and Social Sciences*, 58, 2, P112-P128.

Pel-Littel, R.E., Schuurmans, M.J., Emmelot-Vonk, M.H. and Verhaar, H.J.J. (2009) 'Frailty: defining and measuring of a concept', *JNHA – The Journal of Nutrition, Health and Aging*, 13, 4, 390-4.

Perkin, H. (1990) *The rise of professional society*, London: Routledge.

Phillipson, C., Bernard, M. and Strang, P. (eds) (1986) *Dependency and interdependency in old age: Theoretical perspectives and policy alternatives*, London: Routledge & Kegan Paul.

Pillemer, K. (1985) 'The dangers of dependency: New findings on domestic violence against the elderly', *Social Problems*, 33, 2, 146-58.

Pollitt, C. (1990) *Managerialism and the public services*, Oxford: Basil Blackwell.

Poole, M., Bond, J., Emmett, C., Greener, H., Louw, S.J., Robinson, L. and Hughes, J.C. (2014) 'Going home? An ethnographic study of assessment of capacity and best interests in people with dementia being discharged from hospital', *BMC Geriatrics*, 14, 1, 56.

Post, S. (1995) 'Alzheimer disease and the "then" self', *Kennedy Institute of Ethics Journal*, 5, 4, 307-21.

Post, S.G. (2006) 'Respectare: moral respect for the lives of the deeply forgetful', in J.C. Hughes, S.J. Louw and S.R. Sabat (eds) *Dementia: Mind, meaning, and the person*, New York: Oxford University Press, pp 223-34.

Price, D., Bisdee, D., Daly, T., Livsey, L. and Higgs, P. (2014) 'Financial planning for social care in later life: the "shadow" of fourth age dependency', *Ageing & Society*, 34, 3, 388-410.

Puts, M.T., Lips, P., Ribbe, M.W. and Deeg, D.J. (2005) 'The effect of frailty on residential/nursing home admission in the Netherlands independent of chronic diseases and functional limitations', *European Journal of Ageing*, 2, 4, 264-74.

Puts, M.T., Shekary, N., Widdershoven, G., Heldens, J. and Deeg, D.J. (2009) 'The meaning of frailty according to Dutch older frail and non-frail persons', *Journal of Aging Studies*, 23, 4, 258-66.

Rabheru, K. (2007) 'Disease staging and milestones', *The Canadian Journal of Neurological Sciences*, 34, S1, S62-S66.

Rabold, S. and Goergen, T. (2013) 'Abuse and neglect of older care recipients in domestic settings – results of a survey among nursing staff of home care services in Hanover (Germany)', *Journal of Adult Protection*, 15, 3, 127-40.

Radin, M.J. (1982) 'Property and personhood', *Stanford Law Review*, 34, 5, 957-1015.

Rainbird, H., Munro, A., Holly, L. and Leisten, R. (1999) *The future of work in the public sector: Learning and workplace inequality*, Swindon: Economic and Social Research Council.

Rawls, J. (1985) 'Justice as fairness: political not metaphysical', *Philosophy & Public Affairs*, 14, 3, 223-51.

Raymond, M., Warner, A., Davies, N., Iliffe, S., Manthorpe, J. and Ahmedzhai, S. (2014) 'Palliative care services for people with dementia: a synthesis of the literature reporting the views and experiences of professionals and family carers', *Dementia*, 13, 1, 96-110.

Reher, D.S. (1998) 'Family ties in Western Europe: Persistent contrasts', *Population and Development Review*, 24, 2, 203-34.

Reich, O., Signorell, A. and Busato, A. (2013) 'Place of death and health care utilization for people in the last 6 months of life in Switzerland: a retrospective analysis using administrative data', *BMC Health Services Research*, 13, 1, 116.

Reid, C.E., Moss, S. and Hyman, G. (2005) 'Caregiver reciprocity: The effect of reciprocity, carer self-esteem and motivation on the experience of caregiver burden', *Australian Journal of Psychology*, 57, 3, 186-96.

Reisberg, B., Ferris, S.H., de Leon, J. and Crook, T. (1982) 'The global deterioration scale for assessment of primary degenerative dementia', *American Journal of Psychiatry*, 139, 10, 1136-9.

Ricoeur, P. (1992) *Oneself as another*, Chicago, IL: Chicago University Press.

Riegel, K.F. and Riegel, R.M. (1972) 'Development, drop, and death', *Developmental Psychology*, 6, 306-19.

Robb, B. (1967) *Sans everything: A case to answer*, London: Nelson.

Rockwood, K., Fox, R.A., Stolee, P., Robertson, D. and Beattie, B.L. (1994) 'Frailty in elderly people: an evolving concept', *CMAJ: Canadian Medical Association Journal*, 150, 4, 489-95.

Rockwood, K., Stadnyk, B., MacKnight, C., McDowell, I., Hebert, R. and Hogan, D.B. (1999) 'A brief clinical measure of frailty', *The Lancet*, 353, 205-6.

Rodríguez-Mañas, L., Féart, C., Mann, G., Viña, J., Chatterji, S., Chodzko-Zajko, W., Gonzalez-Colaço, M. and Vega, E. (2013) 'Searching for an operational definition of frailty: a Delphi method-based consensus statement. The frailty operative definition-consensus conference project', *The Journals of Gerontology Series A: Biological Sciences and Medical Sciences*, 68, 1, 62-7.

Rodriguez-Martin, B., Martinez-Andres, M., Cervera-Monteagudo, B., Notario-Pacheco, B. and Martinez-Vizcaino, V. (2014) 'Preconceptions about institutionalisation at public nursing homes in Spain: views of residents and family members', *Ageing & Society*, 34, 4, 547-68.

Rodriquez, J. (2011) '"It's a dignity thing": nursing home care workers' use of emotions', *Sociological Forum*, 26, 2, 265-86.

Rodriquez, J. (2013) 'Narrating dementia: Self and community in an online forum', *Qualitative Health Research*, 23, 9, 1215-27.

Rodriquez, J. (2014) *Labors of love: Nursing homes and the structures of care work*, New York: New York University Press.

Rosen, T., Pillemer, K. and Lachs, M. (2008) 'Resident-to-resident aggression in long-term care facilities: An understudied problem', *Aggression and Violent Behavior*, 13, 2, 77-87.

Rosenthal, D. and Weisberg, J. (2008) 'Higher-order theories of consciousness', *Scholarpedia*, 3, 5, 4407.

Rothman, M.D., Leo-Summers, L. and Gill, T.M. (2008) 'Prognostic significance of potential frailty criteria', *Journal of the American Geriatrics Society*, 56, 12, 2211-16.

Rowe, J.W. and Kahn, R.L. (1987) 'Human aging: usual and successful', *Science*, 237, 4811, 143-9.

Rowland, D.T. (2009) 'Global population aging: History and prospects', in P. Uhlenburg (ed) *International handbook of population aging*, Dordrecht: Springer, pp 37-65.

Rowntree, B.S. (1901) *Poverty: A study of town life*, London: Longmans.

Rowntree, B.S. (1941) *Poverty and progress: A second social survey of York*, London: Longmans, Green & Co.

Rowntree, B.S. and Lavers, G.R. (1954) *Poverty and the welfare state: A third social survey of York*, London: Longmans.

Rushton, N.S. (2001) 'Monastic charitable provision in Tudor England: quantifying and qualifying poor relief in the early sixteenth century', *Continuity and Change*, 16, 1, 9-44.

Sabat, S.R. (2006) 'Mind, meaning, and personhood in dementia: the effects of positioning', in J.C. Hughes, S.J. Louw and S.R. Sabat (eds) *Dementia: Mind, meaning, and the person*, Oxford: Oxford University Press, pp 287-302.

Salter, K., Hellings, C., Foley, N. and Teasell, R. (2008) 'The experience of living with stroke: a qualitative meta-synthesis', *Journal of Rehabilitation Medicine*, 40, 8, 595-602.

Sapontzis, S.F. (1981) 'A critique of personhood', *Ethics*, 91, 607-18.

Sautter, J.M., Tulsky, J.A., Johnson, K.S., Olsen, M.K., Burton-Chase, A.M., Hoff Lindquist, J. et al (2014) 'Caregiver experience during advanced chronic illness and last year of life', *Journal of the American Geriatrics Society*, 62, 6, 1082-90.

Saveman, B.I., Åström, S., Bucht, G. and Norberg, A. (1999) 'Elder abuse in residential settings in Sweden', *Journal of Elder Abuse & Neglect*, 10, 1-2, 43-60.

Schechtman, M. (1994) 'The same and the same: Two views of psychological continuity', *American Philosophical Quarterly*, 31, 3, 199-212.

Schechtman, M. (2003) 'Empathic access: the missing ingredient in personal identity', in R. Martin and J. Barresi (eds) *Personal identity*, Oxford: Blackwell, pp 238-59.

Schoenmakers, B., Buntinx, F. and Delepeleire, J. (2010) 'Factors determining the impact of care-giving on caregivers of elderly patients with dementia. A systematic literature review', *Maturitas*, 66, 2, 191-200.

Schubert, C.C., Boustani, M., Callahan, C.M., Perkins, A.J., Carney, C.P., Fox, C. et al (2006) 'Comorbidity profile of dementia patients in primary care: are they sicker?', *Journal of the American Geriatrics Society*, 54, 1, 104-9.

Searle, S.D., Mitnitski, A., Gahbauer, E.A., Gill, T.M. and Rockwood, K. (2008) 'A standard procedure for creating a frailty index', *BMC Geriatrics*, 8, 1, 24.

Sears, E. (1986) *The ages of man: Medieval interpretations of the life cycle*, Princeton, NJ: Princeton University Press.

Seedhouse, D. and Gallagher, A. (2002) 'Undignifying institutions', *Journal of Medical Ethics*, 28, 6, 368-72.

Sen, A. (1999) *Commodities and capabilities*, New Delhi: Oxford University Press.

Shim, B., Barroso, J., Gilliss, C.L. and Davis, L.L. (2013) 'Finding meaning in caring for a spouse with dementia', *Applied Nursing Research*, 26, 3, 121-26.

Shimada, H., Makizako, H., Doi, T., Yoshida, D., Tsutsumimoto, K., Anan, Y. et al (2013) 'Combined prevalence of frailty and mild cognitive impairment in a population of elderly Japanese people', *Journal of the American Medical Directors Association*, 14, 7, 518-24.

Silverstein, M. and Giarrusso, R. (2010) 'Aging and family life: A decade review', *Journal of Marriage and Family*, 72, 5, 1039-58.

Sims-Gould, J., Byrne, K., Craven, C., Martin-Matthews, A. and Keefe, J. (2010) 'Why I became a home support worker: Recruitment in the home health sector', *Home Health Care Services Quarterly*, 29, 4, 171-94.

Singer P. (1993) *Practical Ethics* 2nd edn, Cambridge: Cambridge University Press.

Sink, K.M., Holden, K.F. and Yaffe, K. (2005) 'Pharmacological treatment of neuropsychiatric symptoms of dementia: a review of the evidence', *JAMA*, 293, 5, 596-608.

Sixsmith, A., Stilwell, J. and Copeland, J. (1993) '"Rementia": challenging the limits of dementia care', *International Journal of Geriatric Psychiatry*, 8, 12, 993-1000.

Skeggs, B. (2011) 'Imagining personhood differently: person value and autonomist working-class value practices', *The Sociological Review*, 59, 3, 498-513.

Smith, C. (2010) *What is a person?*, Chicago, IL: University of Chicago Press.

Smith, G.E., Kokmen, E. and O'Brien, P.C. (2000) 'Risk factors for nursing home placement in a population-based dementia cohort', *Journal of the American Geriatrics Society*, 48, 4, 519-25.

Smith, S.R. (2001) 'Distorted ideals: The "problem of dependency" and the mythology of independent living', *Social Theory and Practice*, 27, 4, 579-98.

Sökefeld, M. (1999) 'Debating self, identity and culture in anthropology', *Current Anthropology*, 40, 4, 417-48.

Somboontanont, W., Sloane, P.D., Floyd, F.J., Holditch-Davis, D., Hogue, C.C. and Mitchell, C.M. (2004) 'Assaultive behavior in Alzheimer's disease: identifying immediate antecedents during bathing', *Journal of Gerontological Nursing*, 30, 9, 22-9.

Sona, A., Zhang, P., Ames, D., Bush, A.I., Lautenschlager, N.T., Martins, R.N. et al (2012) 'Predictors of rapid cognitive decline in Alzheimer's disease: results from the Australian Imaging, Biomarkers and Lifestyle (AIBL) study of ageing', *International Psychogeriatrics*, 24, 2, 197-204.

Sörensen, S. and Conwell, Y. (2011) 'Issues in dementia caregiving: effects on mental and physical health, intervention strategies, and research needs', *The American Journal of Geriatric Psychiatry*, 19, 6, 491-6.

References

St John, P.D., Montgomery, P.R. and Tyas, S.L. (2013) 'Social position and frailty', *Canadian Journal on Aging/La Revue Canadienne du Vieillissement*, 32, 3, 250-9.

Stacey, C.L. (2005) 'Finding dignity in dirty work: the constraints and rewards of low-wage home care labour', *Sociology of Health and Illness*, 27, 6, 831-54.

Stacey, C.L. (2011) *The caring self: The work experiences of home care aides*, New York: Cornell University Press.

Staff, R.T., Chapko, D., Hogan, M. and Whalley, L.J. (2016) 'Life course socioeconomic status and the decline in information processing speed in late life', *Social Science & Medicine*, 151, 130-8.

Stone, R.I. and Wiener, J.M. (2001) *Who will care for us: Addressing the long-term care workforce crisis*, Washington, DC: The Urban Institute and the American Association of Homes and Services for the Ageing (www.urban.org/research/publication/who-will-care-us-addressing-long-term-care-workforce-crisis/view/full_report).

Stone, R.I., Sutton, J.P., Bryant, N., Adams, A. and Squillace, M. (2013) 'The home health workforce: A distinction between worker categories', *Home Health Care Services Quarterly*, 32, 4, 218-33.

Strawbridge, W.J., Wallhagen, M.I. and Cohen, R.D. (2002) 'Successful aging and well-being self-rated compared with Rowe and Kahn', *The Gerontologist*, 42, 6, 727-33.

Strawson, P.E. (1971) *Individuals: An essay in descriptive metaphysics*, London: Methuen University Paperbacks.

Sugarman, J. (2005) 'Persons and moral agency', *Theory & Psychology*, 15, 6, 793-811.

Surr, C.A. (2006) 'Preservation of self in people with dementia living in residential care: A socio-biographical approach', *Social Science & Medicine*, 62, 7, 1720-30.

Suzman, R. and Riley, M.W. (1985) 'Introducing the "oldest-old"', *Milbank Memorial Fund Quarterly*, 63, 177-86.

Swartz, T.T. (2009) 'Intergenerational family relations in adulthood: Patterns, variations, and implications in the contemporary United States', *Annual Review of Sociology*, 35, 191-212.

Sweeting, H. and Gilhooly, M. (1997) 'Dementia and the phenomenon of social death', *Sociology of Health & Illness*, 19, 1, 93-117.

Szanton, S.L., Seplaki, C.L., Thorpe, R.J., Allen, J.K. and Fried, L.P. (2010) 'Socioeconomic status is associated with frailty: the Women's Health and Aging Studies', *Journal of Epidemiology and Community Health*, 64, 1, 63-7.

Tanner, D. (2012) 'Co-research with older people with dementia: experience and reflections', *Journal of Mental Health*, 21, 3, 296-306.

Taylor, C. (1985) 'The person', in M. Carrithers, S. Collins and S. Lukes (eds) *The category of the person: Anthropology, philosophy, history*, Cambridge: Cambridge University Press, pp 257-81.

Taylor, C. (1992) *Sources of the self: The making of the modern identity*, Cambridge: Cambridge University Press.

Themessl-Huber, M., Hubbard, G. and Munro, P. (2007) 'Frail older people's experiences and use of health and social care services', *Journal of Nursing Management*, 15, 2, 222-9.

Theou, O., Brothers, T.D., Mitnitski, A. and Rockwood, K. (2013) 'Operationalization of frailty using eight commonly used scales and comparison of their ability to predict all-cause mortality', *Journal of the American Geriatrics Society*, 61, 9, 1537-51.

Thomas, C. (1993) 'De-constructing concepts of care', *Sociology*, 27, 4, 649-69.

Thomas, C. and Milligan, C. (2015) 'Dementia and the social model of disability', *Joseph Rowntree Viewpoint*, York: Joseph Rowntree Foundation.

Tobin, S.S. and Lieberman, M.A. (1976) *Last Home for the Aged*, San Francisco, CA: Jossey-Bass.

Townsend, P. (1962) *The last refuge: A survey of residential institutions and homes for the aged in England and Wales*, London: Routledge & Kegan Paul.

Townsend, P. (1968) 'Summary and conclusions', in E. Shanas, P. Townsend, D. Wedderburn, H. Friis, P. Milhøj and J. Stehouwer (eds) *Old people in three industrial societies*, London: Routledge & Kegan and Paul, pp 424-53.

Townsend, P. (1981) 'The structured dependency of the elderly: a creation of social policy in the twentieth century', *Ageing and Society*, 1, 1, 5-28.

Tronto, J. (1993) *Moral boundaries: A political argument for an ethic of care*, New York: Routledge.

Tschanz, J.T., Corcoran, C.D., Schwartz, S., Treiber, K., Green, R.C., Norton, M.C. et al (2011) 'Progression of cognitive, functional, and neuropsychiatric symptom domains in a population cohort with Alzheimer dementia: the Cache County Dementia Progression study', *The American Journal of Geriatric Psychiatry*, 19, 6, 532-42.

Turner, B.S. (1986) 'Personhood and citizenship', *Theory, Culture & Society*, 3, 1, 1-16.

Turner, B.S. (2006) *Vulnerability and human rights*, University Park, PA: Pennsylvania State University Press.

Turner, B.S. (2009) *Can we live forever? A sociological and moral inquiry*, London: Anthem Press.

References

Twigg, J. (1992) *Carers: Research and practice*, London: HMSO.

Twigg, J. (2000) 'Carework as a form of bodywork', *Ageing & Society*, 20, 4, 389-411.

Twigg, J., Wolkowitz, C., Cohen, R.L. and Nettleton, S. (2011) 'Conceptualising body work in health and social care', *Sociology of Health & Illness*, 33, 2, 171-88.

Twining, L. (1885) 'State hospitals: Or, nursing in workhouse infirmaries', *Good Words*, 26, 667-70.

UN (United Nations) (2014) *UN world population prospects, 2013*, New York: UN.

Ungerson, C. (2002) 'Care as a commodity', in B. Bytheway, V. Bacigalupo, J. Bornat, J. Johnson and S. Spurr (eds) *Understanding care, welfare and community*, London: Routledge, pp 351-62.

van Delden, J.J.M. (2004) 'The unfeasibility of requests for euthanasia in advance directives', *Journal of Medical Ethics*, 30, 5, 447-51.

Vandervoort, A., van den Block, L., van der Steen, J.T., Volicer, L., Vander Stichele, R., Houttekier, D. and Deliens, L. (2013) 'Nursing home residents dying with dementia in Flanders, Belgium: a nationwide postmortem study on clinical characteristics and quality of dying', *Journal of the American Directors Association*, 14, 7, 485-92.

Vandervoort, A., van den Block, L., van der Steen, J.T., Stichele, Vander, R., Bilsen, J. and Deliens, L. (2012a) 'Advance directives and physicians' orders in nursing home residents with dementia in Flanders, Belgium: prevalence and associated outcomes', *International Psychogeriatrics*, 24, 7, 1133-43.

Vandervoort, A., van den Block, L., van der Steen, J.T., Volicer, L., Stichele, V.R., Collard, R.M. et al (2012b) 'Prevalence of frailty in community-dwelling older persons: A systematic review', *Journal of the American Geriatrics Society*, 60, 8, 1487-92.

van Iersel, M.B. and Rikkert, M.G. (2006) 'Frailty criteria give heterogeneous results when applied in clinical practice', *Journal of the American Geriatric Society*, 54, 4, 728-9.

van Kan, G.A., Rolland, Y., Houles, M., Gillette-Guyonnet, S., Soto, M. and Vellas, B. (2010) 'The assessment of frailty in older adults', *Clinics in Geriatric Medicine*, 26, 2, 275-86.

Veatch, R.M. (1998) 'The place of care in ethical theory', *Journal of Medicine and Philosophy*, 23, 2, 210-24.

Vermeulen, J., Neyens, J.C., van Rossum, E., Spreeuwenberg, M.D. and de Witte, L.P. (2011) 'Predicting ADL disability in community-dwelling elderly people using physical frailty indicators: a systematic review', *BMC Geriatrics*, 11, 1, 33.

Vladeck, B.C. (1980) *Unloving care: The nursing home tragedy*, New York: Basic Books.
von Bonsdorff, M., Rantanen, T., Laukkanen, P., Suutama, T. and Heikkinen, E. (2006) 'Mobility limitations and cognitive deficits as predictors of institutionalization among community-dwelling older people', *Gerontology*, 52, 6, 359-65.
von Kutzleben, M., Schmid, W., Halek, M., Holle, B. and Bartholomeyczik, S. (2012) 'Community-dwelling persons with dementia: What do they need? What do they demand? What do they do? A systematic review on the subjective experiences of persons with dementia', *Aging & Mental Health*, 16, 3, 378-90.
Vygotsky, L. (1978) *Mind in society: The development of higher mental process*, Cambridge, MA: Harvard University Press.
Walker, A. (1980) 'The social creation of poverty and dependency in old age', *Journal of Social Policy*, 9, 1, 49-75.
Walsh, C.A. and Yon, Y. (2012) 'Developing an empirical profile for elder abuse research in Canada', *Journal of Elder Abuse & Neglect*, 24, 2, 104-19.
Wang, D. and Chonody, J. (2013) 'Social workers' attitudes toward older adults: A review of the literature', *Journal of Social Work Education*, 49, 1, 150-72.
Warmoth, K., Lang, I.A., Phoenix, C., Abraham, C.A., Andrews, M.K., Hubbard R.E. and Tarrant, M. (2015) '"Thinking you're old and frail": a qualitative study of frailty in older adults', *Ageing & Society*, doi: 10.1017/S0144686X1500046X.
Webster, C. (1991) 'The elderly and the early national health service', in M. Pelling and R.M. Smith (eds) *Life, death and the elderly: Historical perspectives*, London: Routledge, pp 165-92.
Weidemann, E.J. (2012) 'The ethics of life and death: advance directives and end-of-life decision making in persons with dementia', *Journal of Forensic Psychology Practice*, 12, 1, 81-96.
Wells, Y.D. (1999) 'Intentions to care for a spouse: gender differences in anticipated willingness to care and expected burden', *Journal of Family Studies*, 5, 2, 220-34.
Whitehouse, P.J. (1993) 'Cholinergic therapy in dementia', *Acta Neurologica Scandinavica*, Suppl 149, 42-5.
Whittaker, E. (1992) 'The birth of the anthropological self and its career', *Ethos*, 20, 2, 191-219.
Wiles, J. (2011) 'Reflections on being a recipient of care: Vexing the concept of vulnerability', *Social & Cultural Geography*, 12, 6, 573-88.
Willcocks, D., Peace, S. and Kellaher, L. (1987) *Private lives in public places*, London: Tavistock.

References

Williams, G. (1984) 'The genesis of chronic illness: narrative reconstruction', *Sociology of Health & Illness*, 6, 175-200.

Williams, S.J. (2000) 'Chronic illness as biographical disruption or biographical disruption as chronic illness? Reflections on a core concept', *Sociology of Health & Illness*, 22, 40-67.

Williams, S.J., Higgs, P. and Katz, S. (2012) 'Neuroculture, active ageing and the "older brain": problems, promises and prospects', *Sociology of Health & Illness*, 34, 1, 64-78.

Wolff, J.L. and Agree, E.M. (2004) 'Depression among recipients of informal care: the effects of reciprocity, respect, and adequacy of support', *The Journals of Gerontology Series B: Psychological Sciences and Social Sciences*, 59, 3, S173-S180.

Woo, J., Goggins, W., Sham, A. and Ho, S.C. (2005) 'Social determinants of frailty', *Gerontology*, 51, 402-8.

Woo, J., Leung, J. and Morley, J.E., (2012) Comparison of frailty indicators based on clinical phenotype and the multiple deficit approach in predicting mortality and physical limitation, *Journal of the American Geriatrics Society*, 60(8), 1478-1486.

Woods, A.J., Cohen, R.A. and Pahor, M. (2013) 'Cognitive frailty: Frontiers and challenges', *The Journal of Nutrition, Health & Aging*, 17, 9, 741-8.

Zarit, S.H. (1989) 'Do we need another "stress and caregiving" study?', *The Gerontologist*, 29, 2, 147-8.

Zeller, A., Hahn, S., Needham, I., Kok, G., Dassen, T. and Halfens, R.J. (2009) 'Aggressive behavior of nursing home residents toward caregivers: a systematic literature review', *Geriatric Nursing*, 30, 3, 174-87.

Index

A

abjection 8, 57–72
  concept origins 57–60
  fate of 60–3
  'frailty' as new marker for 63–5
  healthcare work and the 'abject classes' 65–7
  institutionalised abuse 68–70
  occurrences of abuse 67–70
abuse in care settings 67–70, 107–8
accountability and personhood 19–20
advance directives 121–4
advanced infirmity 111–26
  illness trajectories 113–15
  measurement of and narratives for 116–19
  terminal personhood and dementia 119–24
advanced old age 1–2
  demographics 1
  modelling of 2–6
'agency / loss of agency' 9
  in the co-construction of care 84–5
  developmental nature of 22–3
  and frailty 50–1
  measuring stages of decline 116–19
  and personhood 17–19, 119–21
  retaining expressions of 114–15
  structure and reflexivity (Archer) 37–9
  three aspects of (Giddens) 35–6
  use of advance directives 121–4
  vs. narratives of dementia 112, 118–19
'agency-plus' (Taylor) 22–3
Allen, RS et al 123
Alzheimer's disease and agency 89–90
Andersson, I et al 114–15
anthropological concepts of self 33–4
Archer, Margaret 37–9
'at homeness' 105–6

B

Baldwin, C and Capstick, A 132
Baltes, Paul 5–6, 115
Bartlett, R and O'Connor, D 137
Bataille, Georges 60–2
Beckett, Samuel 77
Beck, U 36–7, 43–4, 45, 96
Buber, Martin 13

C

Callegaro, F 28–9
capacity 121–4, 137–8
  and 'entitlement' 138
care
  co-construction of 84–5, 115, 119–21, 125–6
  'deservedness' of treatment 20–1
  identity and agency 82–4
  and the moral imperative 52–4, 77–80, 91–2
  nature of 74–7
  reciprocity and relationships 85–7
  role of personhood 11–26
    morality constructs 19–25, 130–2, 136–7
  seen as 'assault' 69
  as 'service' 104–5
  in the shadow of the fourth age 87–91
  social relations of 80–2
  in terminal 'fourth age' 111–38
care relationships
  adult children and intimations of mortality 83
  in advanced infirmity 87–91
  care home studies 104–5
  and co-construction of care 84–5, 115, 119–21, 125–6
  and 'emotional labour' 99–100, 104–5, 125–6
  and estrangement 69–71, 81–2, 87–8, 92, 102, 110, 113

inter-dependency and abuse 69–70, 107–8
as intrinsic motivation 100–1
moral imperatives of 52–4, 77–80, 91–2, 130–1, 133–4
one-sided nature of 129–30
reciprocity in 85–7, 123–4, 129–30
spousal care and identity 82, 129–30
care work 65–7, 70, 93–110
brief history 95–9
in care homes 103–5
contemporary patterns 99–101
contractual basis of 129–31
dignity and value in 66–7, 106–7
expectations of 107
experiences of 101–3
moral order and ethos of 106–9, 130–1
in own homes 105–6
privileging of feelings and relatedness 135
standards of 108–9
status of 67, 106–7
without 'limits' (in advanced infirmity) 111–26
care workers 99–101, 107–8
'abject' nature of work 65–7, 70
demographics of 99–100
and emotional labour 99–100, 104–5, 125–6
experiences of caring 101–2
as 'moral agents' 26, 100–1, 130–1, 132–3, 137
motivations of 100–1, 133
non-professional discourses 108
pay 99–100
personhood of 136
and professionalisation 107–8
relationship with family members 108
as responsible for 'personhood' of cared for 25, 124–5
'second-order' motives (Frankfurt) of 133
as 'strangers' 69–71, 81–2, 87–8, 92, 102, 110, 113
subordination of 135–6
suffering abuse 69–70, 107–8
Christian tradition of old age relief 3
Clare, L 115, 118, 129
co-constructions of care 115, 119–21, 125–6
cognitive decline 113–15
measurement of 116–19
and 'ownership' of self 121–4
terminal personhood 119–21

'common humanity' of a person 26, 27, 133, 135–6
consciousness
and developmental nature of personhood 23–4
Durkheimmian views 29–30
and experience 14–15
and reflexivity 34–5
and sense of self 30–3
and volition 17–19
The constitution of society (Giddens) 35
Cooley, Charles 30
'cultural field(s) of the third age' (Gilleard and Higgs) 2

D

Dan-Cohen, M 41
Davies, N et al 120
de Boer, ME et al 122
death proximity as fourth age 'marker' 3–4
Degnen, C 7
dementia
fears of 44
and frailty 49, 88–91
impact of individualisation culture 36–7, 135
loss of agency and identity 90–1, 114–15, 119–21, 121–4
mapping and staging 116–19
narrative accounts of 118–19
ownership of self 121–4
and personhood 11–26, 88–90, 119–21
psychopathology of 117–18
quality of life in 120
'social citizenship' discourses 137–8
studies on being cared for 103
terminal personhood of 119–21
trajectories of 89–90, 116–19
dementia and 'stranger–care' 87–91
Dennett, Daniel 18–19, 29
dependency 5–6, 9–10, 46, 52–5, 83
and abuse 67–70
fears of 11
and inter-dependency 107–8
see also advanced infirmity
Déscartes, Rene 14
destitution 58–9
developmental approach to personhood 22–4
dignity and worth in care work 66–7
'dirty work' of care 65–7
and abuse 67–70

174

Index

'disrupted biographical narrative' of illness 114
'dualism of human nature' (Durkheim) 28–9
Durkheim, Emile 28–9, 33, 129
Dwyer, LL *et al* 115

E

'ego identity' (Goffman) 32–3
elder abuse 67–70, 107–8
'embodied personhood' (Turner) 39–40
'emotional authenticity' (Lopez) in care work 104–5
'emotional labour' as evidence of quality care 99–100, 104–5, 125–6
'empathic access' (Schechtman) 17
end-stage care 111–26
  journeys in 113–15
  measurement of 116–19
  and terminal personhood 119–21
  use of advance directives 121–4
England, P 76
Engster, D 76–7
euthanasia 121–4
'extreme individualism' 11–12, 128

F

family care
  and elder abuse 67–8
  identity and ambiguities 82–4
  moral and social values 77–80
  nature of caring 74–7
  parents as 'shield against mortality' 83
  see also care relationships
family members
  and advance care planning 123
  'judging' and being 'judged' 108
Farah, MJ and Heberlain, AS 21
'first-order volitions (Frankfurt) 18–19
Flatt, MA *et al* 4–5
formal care *see* care; care work; institutional settings
formal carers *see* care workers
Foucault, Michel 59
'fourth age' 1–2, 5–6
  modelling of 2–6
  as 'social / cultural imaginary' 6–8, 8–9
'fourth age imaginary' (Higgs and Gilleard) 6–8, 111–12, 133–4, 134–8
  care in 111–26
  elements of 8–9

frailty 45–55
  biomedical models of 46–8
  as compromised agency/flawed identity 50–1
  as cumulative disadvantage 50–1
  entering institutional care 87–91
  experiences of being cared for 103
  and the fourth age imaginary 2–3, 8, 88–9
  as loss of health reserves 48–50
  making use of 52–3
  as marker of the 'abject classes' 63–5
  and the moral imperative of care 52–4
  nature of 89–90
  prevalence demographics of 51
  resistance to/rejection of 52–3
  and 'unsuccessful ageing' 50–1
  without dementia 88
Frankfurt, Harry 18, 133
Fried, LP *et al* 6, 45, 47–9

G

Garcia-Garcia, FJ *et al* 51
Geertz, Clifford 130
Gerstorf, D and Ram, N 4
Giddens, Anthony 34–7
Gilleard, CJ and Higgs, P 2–3, 6–8, 11, 41, 43, 62–3, 73, 119, 124, 133, 134–5
Gilligan, Carole 75
Gobbens, RJ *et al* 50–1
Goffman, Erving 31–3, 68
Goodman, C *et al* 120
Gordijn, B 132
Grenier, A and Hanley, J 52–3

H

Harrison, JK *et al* 117
Hegel, GWF 20
Hennings, J *et al* 119
Hertogh, CM 122
Higgs, P and Gilleard, CJ 7–8, 45, 119, 129, 133
Himmelfarb, G 57–60
Hirsch, C 51
Hirschfeld, M 86
Hirschman, KB *et al* 123
Hochschild, AR 125
Hogan, DB *et al* 47
home-based care facilities 105–6
  see also family care
homo duplex (Durkheim) 129

Human nature and the social order (Cooley) 30
human rights 21
Hume, David 15, 41

I

identity
  and developmental processes of ageing 22–4
  metaphysics and personhood 14–16
  and self/selves 16–17
  and symbolic interactionism 30–3
  and terminal dementia 119–21, 124–5
  volition and reflexivity 17–19
  see also moral identity; personal identity; personhood
'impotent by age' 2, 9, 46, 50–1, 62–5, 70–1, 96–7, 127
independent living 53
individualisation
  autonomy and rationality 11–12, 128
  as structural requirement of contemporary societies 36–7, 128
infants and moral agency 23
infirmity as 'disrupted biography' 114
informal care
  and 'at homeness' 105–6
  identity and agency 82–4
  transfers to formal care 111–12, 113–15
  vs formal care 80–2
  see also family care
institutional settings 103–5
  background history of 57–60
  burdensome nature of care work 65–7, 70
  carer abuse 69–70, 107–8
  conflicts between residents 69
  and elder abuse 67–70
  introducing culture change 109
  power relations 34
  resource levels 69
  and 'stranger care' 87–91
  see also care work; care workers
inter-dependency
  and abuse 68, 107–8
  see also care relationships
inter-generational proximity 78–9

J

Jetten, J *et al* 118

K

Kahn, RL 4
Kant, Immanuel 15, 20, 22
Kitwood, Tom 11–13, 24–6, 36–7, 121, 128–9, 131–3, 135
Korsgaard, CM 17–18
Kristeva, Julia 60

L

Laslett, Peter 1, 5–6, 75–6
Lee, RP *et al* 120
legal rights, and personhood 21
Lewinter, M 86
Locke, John 15
Lopez, SH 105
'lumpen' classes (Marx) 58–9

M

McCarthy, M *et al* 119–20
MacIntyre, Alistair 16
'malign social psychology' (Kitwood) 25, 128, 133
Manthorpe, J 68
Marx, Karl 43, 58–9
material wealth and personhood 40–1
Mauss, Marcel 29–30, 33
Mead, George 28, 30–1
memory 15
mental capacity
  and abjection 63–5
  and advance directives 121–4
  and 'entitlement' 138
  and expressions of agency 114–15, 137–8
  legal concept of 123
  metaphysics and personhood 13–14, 14–16, 19
  vs moral personhood 19–22
Mind, self and society (Mead) 30–1
Mischel, Walter 22
Mitchell, SL *et al* 117
Mitniski, AB *et al* 47, 48–9
Modernity and self-identity (Giddens) 36
Mooney, MA 28
moral agency 19–20, 23–4, 26, 137
  and metaphysical agency (Taylor) 19
moral identity 22, 24–5, 130–1, 137
  of care work 100–1, 110
  developmental nature of personhood 22–4
'the moral imperative of care ' 52–4, 77–80, 91–2, 130–1
moral order of care work 106–9, 130–1

moral status 13–14, 27, 131–2, 136–7
　and consciousness 21
　and personhood 19–22, 24–5
　potential loss of 23–4

N

narratives of ageing, infirmity and care 9, 12, 16–19, 36, 73–4, 111–15, 118–20, 122
A new map of life (Laslett 1989, 1996) 1, 5–6
Nicholson, C *et al* 120
Nietzsche, Friedrich 67
Noddings, Nel 74–5
Norton, MC 87
nursing homes 63
　'care-as-service' 104–5
　see also care work; institutional settings

O

Ohlin, JD 21, 25, 132
older people demographics, income and wealth 62–3
Oneself as another (Ricoeur) 16–18, 118

P

Paley, J 67
Palmore, E and Cleveland, W 3
Parfit, D 16–17, 21
Perring, C 20–1
person-centred care 11–12, 20, 127–8
　as defining care policy and practice 11–12, 127–8, 131–4
　critiques of 131–4
　effectiveness studies 108–9
　and 'malign social psychology' 128
personal identity
　works of Erving Goffman 32–3
　works of Margaret Archer 37–9
　see also identity; personhood
personhood 11–26
　ambivalence of 'person' 13–14, 128–31
　anthropological discourses 33–4
　concept history 13–14
　deconstruction into agency, identity, autonomy and rationality 25–6, 27, 128
　in defining care policy and practice 11–12, 127–8, 131–4
　critique of 131–4

developmental nature of and moral identity 22–4
Durkheimian views 28–30, 129
　and legal rights 21
　as metaphysical identity 14–16
　and moral status 19–22, 24–5
　neuro-scientific basis 21–2
　as (only) social identity 40–1, 41–3
　as 'others' responsibility 25
　persons as agents 17–19
　as property and status 39–41
　relationships and moral solidarity (Kitwood) 12
　and self/selves 16–17
　as a 'status' between persons 124–6
　and structures of power 34
　'thin identity' of (Geertz) 130, 131
　'philosophy of care' informed by a 'fourth age' 133–8
Piaget, J 22
Pillemer, Karl 68
Poole, M *et al* 123
'post-modernisation' care discourses, reflexivity 34–9
poverty
　contemporary accounts of 62–3
　and dependency 57–60
power and structuration of personhood 34
Powers of horror: An essay on objection (Kristeva) 60
'precedent autonomy' 121–2
The presentation of self in everyday life (Goffman) 31–3
Price, D *et al* 124
professionalisation and care workers 107–8
property and personhood 39–41
Puts, MT *et al* 46, 51–2

R

Radin, Margaret 15, 40–1
Rawls, J 52
Raymond, M *et al* 120
reciprocity, and care relationships 85–7
reflexivity 34–9
　and agency 19
　and consciousness 34–5
　and symbolic interactionism 33
　works of Margaret Archer 37–9
Reher, DS 78–9
relationships *see* care relationships
responsibility and self boundaries 41
retirees, relative poverty levels 62–3

Ricoeur, Paul 16–18, 118
'rights-based' concepts of personhood 21–2
Rodriquez, Jason 70, 119, 130–1
Rowe, JW and Kahn, RL 1, 4–5
Rowntree, BS 71

S

Sabat, SR 133
Sapontzis, SF 12, 21
Schechtman, M 16–17
'second modernity' (Beck) 44, 63–4
Seedhouse, D and Gallagher, A 69
'self' 16–17
  anthropological discourses 33–4
  dual nature of (Mauss) 29–30
  Durkheimian views 28–30
  and empathic access (Schechtman) 17
  as 'matters of degree' (Parfit) 16–17
  metaphysics and personhood 14–16
  works of Margaret Archer 37–9
  see also identity; personhood
'selfhood' (Ricoeur) 16
Singer, Peter 138
Skeggs, Beverly 39–40
Smith, C 28
Smith, SR 53
social agency 31, 42, 62, 71
'social beings' (Durkheim) 28–30, 31
'social citizenship' discourses 137–8
social identity as personhood 40–1, 41–3
  see also social agency
social relations of care 80–2
  see also care relationships
social 'selves' (Mead) 30–1
Sökefeld, M 34
spousal relations and informal care 82–3
  and reciprocity 85–7, 129–30
'stages of life' ageing approaches 5–6
status and personhood 39–41
Stigma (Goffman) 32
'stranger-care' 69–71, 81–2, 87–8, 92, 102, 110, 113
Strawson, P.E. 14
'successful' vs 'unsuccessful' ageing 1–2, 4, 50–1
Surr, CA 118
symbolic interactionism and 'self' 30–3
Szanton, SL *et al* 51

T

Taylor, Charles 14, 18–19, 22–3, 25
'terminal decline', theory of, 3–4
Theou, O *et al* 47
'thin identity' of personhood (Geertz) 130, 131
'third age' of ageing 2
Thomas, C 80
Townsend, P 62, 69
'trajectory of the self' (Giddens) 36–7
A treatise of human nature (Hume) 41
Turner, Bryan 39–40

U

'unsuccessful ageing' 1–2, 4, 48–9, 50–1

V

van Delden, JJM 122
Vandervoort, A *et al* 120, 122
Veatch, RM 75
volition and personhood 17–19
  see also 'agency / loss of agency'
voluntary euthanasia 121–4
von Kutzleben, M *et al* 115
Vygotsky, Lev 22, 31

W

Waiting for Godot (Beckett) 77
Warmouth, K *et al* 52
Weidemann, EJ 121–2
Whittaker, Elvi 33
Williams, SJ *et al* 23

Z

Zarit, Steven 74